The Complete Guide to Infertility

Diagnosis, Treatment, Options

Olga B.A. van den Akker

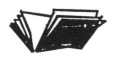

FREE ASSOCIATION BOOKS / LONDON / NEW YORK

First published in Great Britain in 2002 by
FREE ASSOCIATION BOOKS
57 Warren Street
London W1T 5NR

www.fa-b.com

ISBN 1 85343 540 6 pbk

A CIP catalogue record for this book is available from the British Library

Reprints: 10   9   8   7   6   5   4   3   2   1   0

Designed and produced for Free Association Books by
Chase Publishing Services, Fortescue, Sidmouth EX10 9QG
Printed in the European Union by Antony Rowe, Chippenham, England

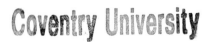

This book is dedicated to my parents,
Boudina and Jacobus van den Akker

Contents

List of Tables

List of Figures

Acknowledgements

I would like to thank everyone who has participated in all my previous research. They have shown me how little information they have had, and how much they needed. I also would like to acknowledge Professor Richard Lilford for giving me creative freedom, Professor Keith Phillips for giving me consideration and confidence, and my children, Max, Basje and Olivia, for giving me understanding and space for 'being busy'.

Preface

There is probably nothing more interesting, more complicated and more meaningful than the human reproductive system. It interacts with all other systems, including the mind, and with what are or will become other beings. The reproductive system gives us psychological meaning, a social and cultural role, physiological pleasure and discomfort, and, if it works adequately, a chance to become the parent of a child. When the reproductive system is challenged, it can affect the meaning of our existence, our perceived role in society, our perception of its pleasures and pain; and can lead us to believe we are infertile.

My goal in writing his book is to engage readers' interest in a field where knowledge and advances progress rapidly. This text does not just provide background information, but provides essential reading for those who wish to increase their knowledge beyond what is provided here. The book is organised into easy-to-read chapters which build on each other, although each can be read on its own. Key words appear in bold and these are explained in an extensive glossary.

The book aims to inform fertile and more particularly infertile people as well as some professionals in areas of nursing, midwifery, psychology, counselling, sociology, social work, social policy and ethics, and their students. For professionals hampered by the limitations of their specialism, this guide provides essential background information to all alternative options available, and the processes involved in each. For those wishing to have a child, knowledge about the relevant systems and their functions is often incomplete. If individuals are well informed at the start of their route through diagnosis and treatments for infertility, with a good basic understanding of the reproductive system, sex, history-taking, diagnosis and finally treatment and the possible psychological effects, then they are prepared in advance for the challenges to be faced. Furthermore, they will be well informed about *all* the options available to them, not just those available within their particular treatment centre. This, hopefully unbiased, account of currently available options and their effects on those using them is therefore intended to provide information for anyone seeking to overcome childless-ness and for the professionals involved in their care. All the options available are included in this guide. Ethical concerns regarding the wider implications of the use of these alternative options to overcome infertility are also discussed in some depth.

Introduction

The World Health Organization (WHO, 1992) reported nearly a decade ago that up to 10% of couples were unable to conceive, and a further 10–25% were unable to have a second or subsequent child (Khanna et al., 1992). Within the UK, estimates are that one in six couples is infertile (Kon, 1993). The infertile therefore constitute a large proportion of our population, many of whom want to seek treatment to overcome this often unwanted condition. Childlessness is not in itself a life-threatening illness, and treatment considerations reflect this. However, people deserve help to overcome this condition, if they believe that having a child would enhance their lives.

Over the years, infertility has shifted from being considered a 'private' problem to a 'public' problem of social concern. The public construction of this social concern has led to controversies in debates over infertility as a problem requiring high-tech treatments, and infertility as a socially constructed illness. The arduous nature of the diagnostic and treatment procedures, and the social stigma and psychological scarring that may follow the diagnosis of infertility, suggests that care and assistance is needed for infertile populations, in clinical treatment, in services and in social psychological terms. On 5 May 1997 a court in Chicago ruled that infertility fits the public definition of a disability, and is therefore subject to the anti-discrimination enforcement under the Americans with Disabilities Act (cited in Bron and Salmon, 1998). The implications of this are not yet fully known, but the fact that services should be provided and managed properly and unequivocally must be regarded as a step in the right direction.

The enormous progress in scientific developments for reproductive health over the last two decades has brought with it some major reports by government-appointed panels across the world, including the Warnock Report (1984) in the UK and the Waller Report (1984) in Australia. Although society at large appears to be in favour of new techniques for reproduction, they are not altogether comfortable about the implications of their use. Consequently, regulation is often asked for and implemented. The UK boasts a system of care which has been described as superior to that found in the US (White, 1998).

UK regulations address clear licensing of treatment centres, reassuring consumers of the system that all that can be done to protect them is being done, and providing the consumer with peace of mind. Regulation brings with it public discussion, and in the case of assisted conception, decisions have to be faced about aspects of reproduction previously not considered relevant: parenthood and the family, identity, legitimacy and lineage all take on different meanings when far-reaching reproductive technologies are used. Ultimately, the most important aspect to consider is the effect of these technologies on the children born from them. With these philosophical, moral, ethical, legal, psychological and social effects in mind, the following chapters discuss the possibilities available to those who are infertile and wish to overcome childlessness.

This book should help individuals to understand the processes involved in solving the problems faced in combating infertility. An effort is made to explain the complexity of infertility and the terminology used. Some of the voluminous research available is cited in this book, in particular with professional readers in mind. All too often people in one profession are limited by knowledge within their own specialist area. This book gives professionals, students and the general reader with an interest in infertility an insight into functions and dysfunctions within reproductive systems. The social and psychological effects these may have and what can be expected when help is first sought are described in detail. The procedures involved in history-taking, diagnosis and treatment are outlined. The book expands on the usual areas covered by incorporating chapters discussing clinical/technological treatments and alternative options such as surrogacy, adoption and fostering.

As with any condition, infertility can take its toll on one or both partners, and the processes involved in diagnosis and treatment can add even more stress to one or both partners. These burdens are well recognised, and are generally addressed as part of the procedure. However, additional help from experienced counsellors is generally available in the area of infertility, and these issues also are addressed in this book. As a result of the psychosocial effects of infertility and the stresses, strains and financial burdens, an abundance of psychosocial research into infertility has been carried out, including evidence-based pointers for good or improved future practice; the interactive effects of psychological and social systems with the physical systems, and the well-being of any subsequent children. However, the range of topics addressed in infertility research varies as much as the people studied. Researchers have attempted to test hypotheses related to psychogenic causes of infertility (Christie, 1998), the motives of infertile mothers who want to become parents (Colpin et al., 1998), and attempts to cure infertility with psychological treatments (Bardwick, 1974). Not all research is methodologically sound and not all explorations or interpretations are reasonable, yet the majority of work provides a network of insights designed to benefit the infertile.

Individuals who have been unable to conceive naturally may wonder technically why this is so, why it has happened to them, and what can be done about it. Numerous physical and psychological or social problems can result from unwanted childlessness, and many of these problems are dealt with in this book. Health care management and services would also benefit from an understanding of the reasoning behind help-seeking behaviour for primary and secondary infertility. It is possible that culturally determined differences influence these decisions (Olsen et al., 1998) and that the availability of health services also plays a role. Van Balen and Gerrits (2001) point out that the consequences of childlessness are perceived as more negative in developing countries. This inequity is further compounded by the fact that resource-poor areas do not have the material resources and appropriate skills necessary in the use of new reproductive technologies to meet the population needs. Within continents, differences have also been observed. An American population survey between 1982 and 1995 indicated that the increase in infertility during that time period was because of the baby-boom population maturing and their delay in childbearing across many age, parity, marital, race, ethnic and economic status groups (Chandra and Stephen, 1998). They also found that women who sought help for this tended to be married, older and of higher income than those who had not sought help for their infertility. This book aims to provide information on the causes, diagnosis and treatments available today, so that the wider implications of all forms of diagnosis and treatment, and their costs, benefits and limitations, can be understood. Moral and ethical issues run through all aspects of infertility, and hence these are discussed at some length in Chapter 11, to increase understanding of the current and future implications. Legal aspects of infertility are extensive, but are mentioned only briefly in this book in those areas where they are at the forefront.

A further aim of the book is to provide information for those with an interest in reproduction, and thus many of the functions and systems operating adequately or incorrectly are discussed. Llewellyn et al.'s (1997) introduction to reproductive health (their focus is on women's reproductive health) states that

> The childbearing years are a time of increased risk for onset of depression in women. Pregnancy, miscarriage or pregnancy loss, infertility and the postpartum period may challenge a woman's mental health. Virtually no life event rivals the neuroendocrine and psychosocial changes associated with pregnancy and childbirth.

Good health and happiness are also relevant to reproduction. The welfare of infertile individuals must be foremost in everyone's mind. Recent developments in the implementation in the UK (October 2000) of the Human Rights Act (1998) will undoubtedly affect issues of 'reproductive rights'. It is predicted that the Convention rights will impact on National Health Service (NHS) practice and interpretations of the Human Fertilisation and Embryology Authority (HFEA) Act and its Code of Practice (Bahadur, 2001). Blank (1990), in an earlier publication, challenged the issues of 'rights'. He suggests that safe and effective treatments are important considerations in infertility, and should not be secondary issues after the question of access to these treatments. He states that in vitro fertilization (IVF) in particular and other techniques in general have gone through tremendous change from experimental to therapy status, despite evidence which suggests that a high degree of caution should be exercised. This may be seen as contrary to many others' points of view; however, Blank's conclusion that 'resources might be better directed toward prevention of fertility problems and discovering the causes of infertility' should not be underestimated.

1 The Human Reproductive System

There is probably nothing more desirable than 'being normal'; particularly so in reproductive terms. Reproduction is associated with fertility, sexuality, a social way of being, and it provides us with a cultural and biological heritage. Yet the reproductive system is elaborate and complex, and 'normality' cannot be assumed or obtained because it does not exist. Perhaps the thing that makes us as sentient beings so interesting is the fact that we are all similar yet so different. In other words, it is the variations, within limits, that assert us as normal. Normality is defined as conformity to a mean or an average of the occurrence of something we are considering, whether we are talking about the length of our nose or a particular **neuroendocrine** substance that is measurable. Otherwise it is a meaningless term, and grossly misused in our everyday language.

Human reproductive functioning is both observable and to a large extent measurable; that is, individual functions and processes can be quantified. In addition the interplay and interactions between the different functions can be observed and measured. As a result we can say that one substance or an organ is relatively within the normal limits or deviates somewhat or significantly from that norm. Science today often but not always allows us to alter systems, processes and the effects of interactions between these variables. When natural attempts to conceive are exhausted or simply not applicable, we can overcome more serious reproductive obstacles using alternative and at times obvious as well as ingenious technological means to achieve what our reproductive system did not allow us to achieve.

The human reproductive system is made up of many systems involving organs and **glands**, and in order for it to function for reproductive purposes, adequate development and functioning of virtually every system, organ and gland is necessary. For example, in human development, we are born with 23 pairs of **chromosomes**: 22 pairs are non-sex-related and are called **autosomes**; the remaining pair, the sex chromosomes, are differentiated by two X chromosomes in the female, and one X and one Y chromosome in the male.

These are necessary for normal sex-differentiated development and to achieve conception.

Conception for many is not always desirable, and contraception, or science, allows us to plan when *not* to be reproductively active. It does not, however, allow us to plan when to be reproductively active in all cases. In order to see what science can do to assist in achieving reproductive capacity when we ask for it, we must first look at what is necessary to achieve conception. Hence this chapter on the human reproductive system will outline what, in observable and measurable terms, is necessary in order to reproduce.

THE FEMALE REPRODUCTIVE SYSTEM

The organs involved in reproduction are many and varied. Figure 1.1 shows the anatomy of the female reproductive organs.

As can be seen from Figure 1.1, the external genitals or genitalia and other structures cover the **perineum** and the whole area is called the **vulva**. The vulva includes the **mons pubis** (veneris), the **clitoris**, the urethral orifice, the vestibule, the **labia majora** and **minora** and the vaginal orifice. Between the vulva and the anus there is an area called the gynaecological perineum. All these organs are relatively easily observable from the exterior. The mons pubis is the rather fatty pad of tissue above the pubis and is covered by the skin and pubic hair. The labia are the folds of skin and fat which run from the mons to the perineum. In fact the labium has the same embryological origin and is similar in structure and position to the scrotum in the male, as discussed later. The clitoris occupies more or less the same position and is formed in a similar way to the penis, with a rich blood supply and spongy erectile tissue. In comparison to the penis the clitoris is of course tiny. During sexual excitement, the erectile tissue of the **bulb of the vestibule** (which lies beneath the skin on either side of the vagina) becomes swollen or inflated and the glands secrete a mucoid discharge which acts as a lubricant. The vulva is the vaginal opening which leads to the vagina. The **vagina** consists of a length of muscle leading from the vestibule to the **cervix**. The cervix is divided into the external and internal os, and is relatively small (a couple of centimetres). The cervix secretes an alkaline substance which helps sperm to enter the uterus.

Once the uterus has an implanted **embryo**, the cervix acts as a sphincter, or closing mechanism, separating the womb from the vagina. The **womb** or **uterus** is where the growth and further development of a fertilised egg takes place. It is a hollow area consisting

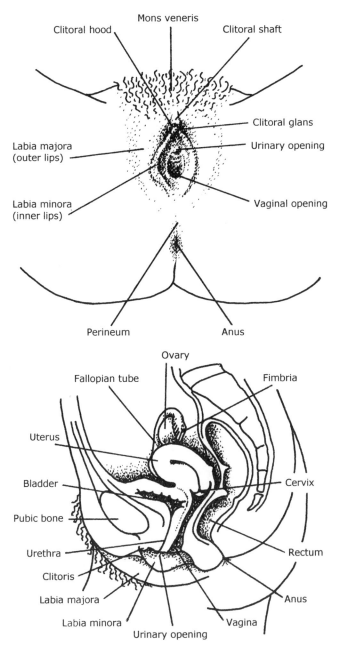

Figure 1.1   The female reproductive system

of muscle, called the **endometrium**. Seen from the inside, it lies between the rectum and the bladder, and is an extension of, or continuous with, the vagina. The endometrium, also called the epithelium, or lining of the uterine 'wall', has a rich blood supply and glands which secrete a small amount of mucus to maintain moistness. The lining of the uterine wall is discarded during **menses**, and this is called **menstruation** or 'periods'. From there we reach the **fallopian tubes**, roughly placed at the top two sides of the inverted triangular womb. The fallopian tubes are thin and about 10 cm long and provide the passage for the ovum into the uterus. The fallopian tubes are mobile to help the ovum towards peristalsis (the muscular movements of contractions and relaxation by which the ovum is moved forward). The reason they are relatively long is to allow enough time for the ovum to mature after it has been fertilised, and before it is ready to implant into the uterus. The fallopian tubes and the **ovaries** are jointly called the adnexae, which means 'parts attached' to the uterus. The end part of the fallopian tube is called the **infundibulum**, which is 2 cm long, expanding at the end. They have **fimbriae** attached at the end to attract or 'catch' the **ovum** or egg, upon maturation from the ovaries.

The ovaries themselves are about 3 cm long and produce and store the ova. Most women are born with about 100,000 ova, which are depleted during each menstrual period and with each pregnancy. Of course, since there are so many thousands of these ova, women never actually run out, but the point is that a woman is born with a finite number of these, whereas a man produces new sperm all the time. In fact more than half the oocytes are internally absorbed before puberty, and all are gone by the time **menopause** is reached. The **corpus luteum** (or 'yellow body') is found in the ovary after rupture of the **graafian follicles** and is derived from the **granulosa** and **theca cells**. During initial growth the graafian follicle moves towards the surface of the ovary and forces the ovum out through the **stigma** and into the waiting fimbriae of the fallopian tube. The follicular cells then become luteinised by the retention of fluid to form the corpus luteum, which in turn secretes **progestins** (hormones) and prepares the uterus for implantation of the fertilised ovum. All other adequate functioning depends on the interactions between many other systems. For example, apart from normal growth, the appearance of the genital tract depends entirely on the supply of the hormone class called **oestrogens**. The very important endocrine system is discussed later.

The female reproductive system therefore works as a magnificent machine, with one part leading to the other through sphincters, fimbriae, peristaltic movements, lubricated tubes, and so on. Each and every action is entirely dependent on the mechanisms needed to initiate, release, transport, catch and maintain the minuscule cargoes. It is surprising that we are barely aware of these events as they take place continuously, with the exception of menstruation and, in some women, ovulation. The way the female reproductive system has evolved therefore requires a certain amount of precision regarding the working together of the anatomical parts and other systems impacting upon them (discussed in later chapters). Nevertheless, there is a fair amount of variation between women in shape and size of the organs involved, and in the amount of contributing effort in related systems, affecting their healthy functioning.

THE MALE REPRODUCTIVE SYSTEM

In the male reproductive system, a **penis** with tubes leading from the **scrotum** and bladder allows the transportation of the **ejaculate**. The ejaculate, the material expelled during **ejaculation**, is produced within the **testes** or **testicles**, and in part as a result of the adrenal gland. As with the woman's reproductive organs, it is important to outline the development of the male genital and reproductive organs because of the so-called anomalies which can occur as a result of organisational defects, endocrine influences or genetic abnormalities. Figure 1.2 shows the anatomy of the male reproductive system.

The penis is both the sex and urinary organ of the male. It becomes enlarged or erect (hence the term **erection**) as a result of the engorgement of the hollow spaces within its substance. The root of the penis is the part attached in the perineum. The testicles lie immediately below the penis and are also attached to the perineum. This is the place where the **spermatozoa** develop. The individual testes are the male **gonads** hanging in the scrotum by the spermatic cord. There is no limit to the production of sperm, unlike the ova supplied by the female.

The male reproductive system looks a lot less complicated than that of the female, and it is. First, the male reproductive system has evolved to deal with fewer aspects of reproduction than the female reproductive system. For example, the male does not possess an area to prepare and maintain in an adequate state for **conception**, **gestation** or delivery of a baby. In essence, all the male does is to

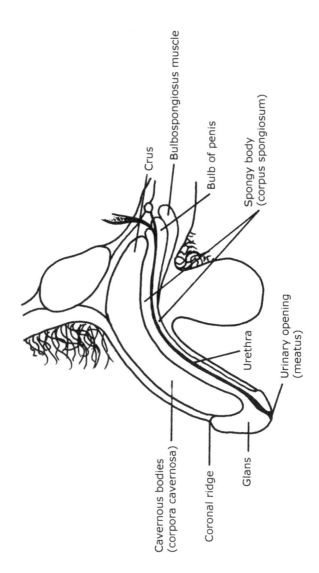

Figure 1.2(a)   The anatomy of the male reproductive system

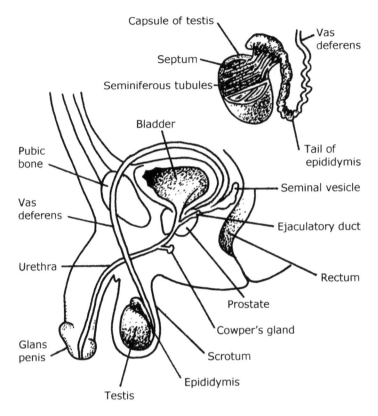

Figure 1.2(b)   The male reproductive system

provide the **gametes** necessary for reproduction. Nevertheless, it is essential that this system too is finely tuned in its production and transportation of sperm and in its interaction with other systems.

HORMONES

Once we know all the organs are in place, and that the tubes actually lead from one place to the next without blockages or leakages, we know the reproductive organs are apparently capable of functioning for reproductive purposes. However, we then need to consider the release and growth of **hormones** through the accompanying glands which make up the **endocrine system**. Each hormone is produced within certain limitations to activate, support, initiate or inhibit other functions. It is therefore extremely important that these are also considered as part of the reproductive system.

Table 1.1 Hormones relevant to the reproductive system

Hormone/endocrine substance	Location/production	Effect/target
Progestins	Ovary	Maintenance of sexually reproductive function
Oestrogens	Ovary	Maintenance of sexually reproductive function
Follicle stimulating hormone (FSH)		Provoke the ovary into producing an ovum
		Formation of the corpus lutum
Luteneising hormone (LH)		
Prolactin	Anterior pituitary	Breast development
Testosterone	Testes	Maintenance of sexually reproductive function
		Enhance the production of spermatozoa in the testes
Growth hormone	Anterior pituitary	Increase in body size
Thyroid stimulating hormone	Anterior pituitary	Enhance metabolism
Adrenocorticotropic hormone (ACTH)	Anterior pituitary	Response to physical stress
Gonadotropic hormones	Anterior pituitary	Growth of gonads or sex glands
Parathormone	Parathyroids	Calcium uptake by bones
Insulin	Pancreas	Glucose uptake by cells

In order to simplify the origins and functions of the hormones needed for a healthy reproductive system, Table 1.1 summarises each one in relation to the female and male reproductive system. Hormones are complex chemical substances secreted by ductless or endocrine glands. They serve as blood-based messengers which regulate cell function in other parts of the body. They can be seen as a large communications network, able to bring about major changes in cell activity. The most dramatic example of the tremendous influence hormones can have is in the pubertal years of an adolescent. Here, in the space of months or years, a child's body undergoes physical processes which transform him or her into a sexually mature young adult. This transformation is the result of the influence of growth and sex hormones. Similarly, if there is a deficiency in a particular hormone whereby growth or development is arrested, therapy with hormones may be able to overcome the disorder caused by the deficiency. The endocrine system functions in close collaboration with the nervous system, and the hypothalamus within the **central nervous system** plays a particularly important role in controlling hormone secretion. The opposite is equally true, where hormones can alter neural function. Figure 1.3 shows the location in the body of all the major endocrine glands which produce the body's hormones. A complex interplay between hormonal secretions and uptake is necessary for the healthy functioning of the reproductive system.

Once we look at the possibility of reproduction and the equipment and ingredients that are necessary to achieve reproduction, it is probably not surprising to anyone that in a good few cases one or more of these systems, functions, organs or glands may not be functioning in an apparently 'normal' (within limits) range or manner.

It is in these cases that it may be necessary to obtain an accurate diagnosis for the lack of fertility or reproductive capacity experienced. This is called 'infertility'. Chapter 3 describes some of the many ways in which a person may experience infertility. However, prior to that it is necessary to understand something about sex. In order to reproduce naturally, sex is necessary. However, even at this stage of reproductive involvement some aspects of sexual functioning may pose obstacles to the possibility of conception. Chapter 2 therefore discusses aspects of sex and sexuality and covers sexual functioning and dysfunctioning to illustrate how **bio-behavioural** systems can also affect reproduction.

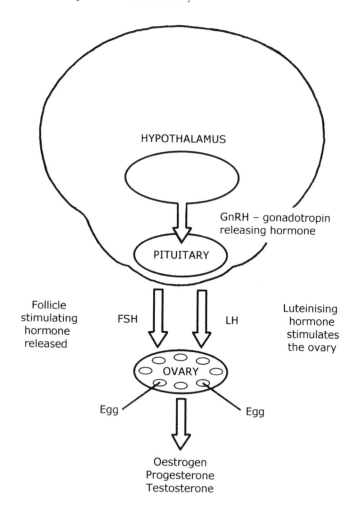

Figure 1.3   The endocrine system

2   Sex and Sexuality

Sex to the majority of people is a private intimate activity which is not discussed openly. This, in a way, is surprising, considering it can enrich people's lives and is considered an important barometer of general health and quality of life. Different cultures acknowledge sex differently, and sexuality in many cultures is linked to femininity, masculinity and reproduction.

In clinical practice, professionals need to consider the importance of sex within the patients' relationship, and this can be difficult for them. O'Gorman et al. (1997) reported on a study assessing communication skills of fifth-year medical students in Ireland. They found that generally they could communicate well about **obstetrics**, **gynaecology** and **genitourinary** medicine, but the majority of medical students had difficulties in talking about sex with their patients, despite the availability of specialist courses on the subject as part of their general training.

The concepts and cultural expression of sex and sexuality have changed over time, from an open and frank display of desire, practise and verbalisation of sex, to the secrecy and repression cultivated by the Victorian bourgeoisie (Foucault, 1976). We are still at the mercy of repressed attitudes towards sex, and consequently we find it difficult to talk about sex. However, if, for the moment at least, we accept that sex is pleasurable, that most of us do it and that it is necessary if reproduction is desired, perhaps talking about it is possible. The study by O'Gorman et al. demonstrates the unequivocal problems our culturally accepted repressions create, even in clinical practice. It is useful to consider these issues when seeking help for infertility because sexual organs and sexual practices will be scrutinised, and both the clinician and the patient need to be able to deal with this.

There are many examples telling of the discomfort felt by men when handing their sperm samples over to nurses, and of women feeling exposed on the examination table (for example, Benson and Robinson-Walsh, 1998, p110). Yet this is the reality of combining sexuality with assistance for clinical conception. Both are necessary, and neither is wrong. Perhaps some frank discussion about sexuality, without going through the discourses unravelled by Foucault, could redress people's attitudes to sex, at least whilst going through assisted conception.

Sexual functioning is a widely researched and written about area. In Chapter 1 the reproductive systems were described, and now a brief mention of sexual functioning seems appropriate since without sex no 'natural' conception can take place. It is fair to assume that most males and females have sex. However, how they have sex, and how often, is related to reproduction. Estimates of sexual **dysfunction** range from 50% of married couples in the US (Masters and Johnson, 1970), to one in ten in the UK (Bancroft, 1983). Sex is important for physical and mental health. When sex is impaired, and one partner has either lost interest or is unable to function sexually, the effects can be marked. Depression, emotional liability, unhappiness and social withdrawal can all result from sexual dysfunction.

It is also important to have some knowledge of sexual behaviour in order to understand what may be regarded as 'abnormal'. Masters et al. (1992) start their substantial edition of human sexuality with a very basic premise: 'Every person has sexual feelings, attitudes and beliefs, but everyone's experience of sexuality is unique because it is processed through an intensely personal perspective.' These prolific writers and investigators about sex explain that being well informed about sex serves many functions, including the prevention of sexual problems. Furthermore, information or education allows the individual to deal effectively with problems. It is worth reiterating what these authors see as different types of sex. According to Masters et al. there are three types of sex: procreational, recreational and relational. This book describes some aspects of sexual behaviour because all three types are relevant to infertility. It is important to understand that the three types of sex will overlap, but at times only sex for recreation or relational purposes will predominate, while at other times – for example, during diagnosis or specific types of treatment – sex for procreation will predominate. The fact that this is seen at times as mechanical could take a back seat if it is accepted that having sex for one reason does not mean that having sex for other reasons is not also possible.

SEXUAL FUNCTION

Sexual behaviour can be divided into a number of different phases, outlined in Figure 2.1. The phases range from initial desire or interest through to arousal or excitement, **orgasm** and finally resolution.

These phases normally follow each other in this order. Most of the behaviour during these phases comes about through visual, tactile, olfactory and mental or perceptual components, though the adequate functioning of some hormones is also necessary. Not much is straightforward in the understanding of the differential effects of different hormones on the sexual behaviour of humans, but what is known is that **androgens** are necessary for the development of full sexual functioning in men and appear to be relevant with respect to women's sex drive. In women, **oestrogens** appear to help in the normal vaginal response to sexual stimulation.

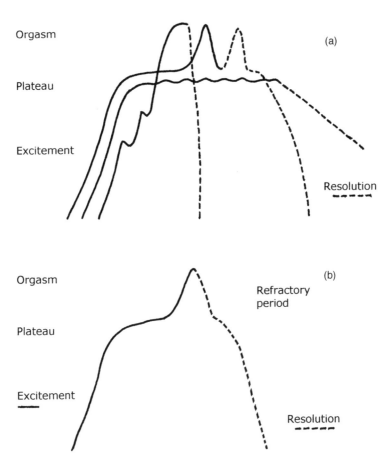

Figure 2.1   Phases during sexual behaviour: female (a) and male (b)

There are a number of signs of sexual excitement. Of course, not all people follow the same responses or patterns. For some, aspects of these may never be present, but Table 2.1 shows generally what happens to women and men when they become sexually excited.

Table 2.1   Female and male sexual excitement signs

Female	Male
Lubrication	Erection of penis (increase in size and
Expansion of the inner two-thirds	firmness)
of the vagina	Skin ridges of scrotum smooth out
Cervix and uterus are pulled forward	Testicles are partially drawn towards
Outer lips of the vagina flatten	body
and move apart	Testes increase slightly in size
Inner lips of vagina enlarge	Nipples become erect
Clitoris increases in size	
Nipples become erect	

In order for the body to respond to sexual excitement a number of systems need to be involved appropriately. The endocrine system works in conjunction with the neuromuscular and vascular systems. Other systems affecting particularly human sexual functioning are the sensory systems and the cognitive systems. Sensory systems refer to olfactory (smell), visual and tactile (touch) processes. Cognitive systems refer to the individual's mental processing and interpretation of the sensory and physiological input. A combination of these helps to achieve sexual stimulation for normal sexual functioning.

SEXUAL DYSFUNCTION

There is a thin line between sexual functioning and dysfunctioning. The majority of sexually active couples will function perfectly normally sexually for most of their sexually active life. For many others, however, different forms of sexual dysfunction can be experienced at one time or another during their sexually active lives. Dysfunction can be mild or severe. In mild cases, sexual dysfunctioning could constitute something as common as lack of desire for weeks or months on end. This can be the result of depression, childbirth followed by exhaustion, drugs, stress at work or hormonal imbalances. In more severe cases, it could be the result of discomfort or even pain, or inability to become sexually **aroused**, as in impotence; or it could be the result of lack of knowledge about sex and sexual behaviour. For these reasons, a discussion of sexual dysfunction is included here.

Since in infertility the focus is on the reproductive organs, and the reproductive organs are also those involved in sex and sexuality, it is inevitable that some adjustment on the part of the individual investigated is necessary. Being closely examined in the morning by a specialist and having those same areas exposed for sex in the evening may cause a mismatch of emotions in many people. This is only to be expected, and with recognition of these difficulties half the problems can be solved. If this is not possible, specific sexual counselling can be obtained, and most clinics should be able to refer an individual or couple for such counselling.

Sexual dysfunction is commonly described according to four main categories: lifelong, acquired, generalised and situational. These speak for themselves, but Table 2.2 summarises them and their explanations. Dysfunction may be the result of psychological causes or stresses, or medical/organic causes. Often it may be a combination of the two. In addition, individual differences in interpretation of function, sexuality, femininity, masculinity and fertility associated with sex or sexuality vary a great deal. Such individual differences must always be borne in mind.

Table 2.2   Types of sexual dysfunction

Type	Description
Lifelong	The problem has been there from the start of sexual behaviour
Acquired	The problem develops after a period of normal functioning
Generalised	The problem is not specific, but is present regardless of type of stimulation, situation or partner(s)
Situational	The problem is specific to certain types of stimulation, situation or partner(s)

Many sexual dysfunctions are well documented, particularly in the medical and psychiatric literature. They can be divided into disorders of arousal, orgasm, lack of control, pain, and other. Arousal dysfunction can be a problem in either the male or the female. In women, this is called **sexual arousal disorder**, and it refers to an inability to obtain or maintain an adequate amount of lubrication-swelling response of sexual excitement. In males, it is called an **erectile disorder**, meaning an inability to obtain or maintain an adequate erection. Arousal problems can occur in either or both partners who are undergoing investigations for fertility. This may be because of the challenge this poses to their sexuality, their fear of failure (particularly noted in men) or because they are focusing their sexual activity entirely on attempts to conceive.

Orgasmic problems in the female and male refer to exactly the same thing. **Female orgasmic disorder** and **male orgasmic disorder** mean a persistent or recurrent delay or an absence of orgasm altogether following normal sexual excitement. **Premature ejaculation** is a condition which involves more of a control problem – the man ejaculates with minimal sexual stimulation before, during or immediately after penetration. This is before the man wishes it to happen, and when he is unable to prevent ejaculation taking place. **Impotence** in men prevents them from being able to have sex because of an inability to achieve an erection. Sexual pain, or dyspareunia, can occur in both men and women and refers to pain before, during or after sex. **Vaginismus** is another condition which can be painful if not recognised. Vaginismus occurs only in women and is characterised by a recurrent or persistent involuntary spasm of the vaginal muscles. The spasm can either prevent sex or interfere with it. Another condition peculiar to women is **sexual aversion disorder**. Women with this condition have a strong aversion to genital contact. Aversion therapy and further consultations with sex therapists can help with many of these problems.

To disclose a sexual problem or concerns about a problem takes a lot of bravery. Most people still do not talk freely about sex, and they are even less likely to discuss any problems or perceived abnormalities in themselves or their partner(s). Similarly, if any one person is already undergoing infertility treatment, this may not be the best time to have a sexual dysfunction investigated. It may be better to leave such an investigation until fertility treatment is completed – unless, of course, it is a dysfunction that is affecting natural conception.

One way for individuals to familiarise themselves with sexual functions and dysfunctions is to read up on sex and sexual activity. Some education about the reproductive system can also be helpful. What is perhaps most crucial is to acknowledge variation, which can help to normalise our behaviour, whether sexual or not. Some individuals will function perfectly adequately sexually until they enter a fertility clinic. In these cases, they may be responding to the stresses involved in the investigations, diagnosis or treatment, and intervention is usually needed when this occurs. It is not within the scope of this book to discuss the procedures involved in sex therapy: suffice it to say that it is essentially a combination of behavioural, psychodynamic and medical interventions, with differing emphasis depending on the dysfunction or issues under investigation.

Psychological effects of infertility have been well documented and will be discussed in Chapter 3, but there are also sexual effects following infertility which need to be considered. In a report on people with normal sexual relations prior to diagnosis, Rosenfeld and Mitchell (1979) observed orgasmic dysfunction and impotence after diagnosis of infertility. In another study, Berger (1980) found that men with male factor infertility were likely to develop impotence following their diagnosis. The fact that these problems have been reported simply shows that professionals have an interest in people's overall well-being, and that in some cases problems can arise following diagnosis or treatment for infertility, not just prior to diagnosis. However, the majority of people under investigation or treatment show no ill-effects on their sexual relationships, behaviour or enjoyment as a result.

Having covered the anatomy and (sexual) behaviour necessary to conceive naturally, the next chapter discusses the incidence, causes and effects of infertility.

FURTHER INFORMATION

Below are some useful services for further information on sexual dysfunction.

Impotence Association
PO Box 10296
London SW17 9WH
www.impotence.org.uk

Information Centre
The Centre for Safe Sex
PO Box 153
Epsom KT18 5WA
Fax: 01372 749 266
www.safe-sex.co.uk

3 Infertility

It is reported that the numbers of people wishing to have children but being unable to have them by spontaneous means is increasing. Infertility can lead to despair for many couples. The first step for most couples is to consult their General Practitioner (GP), who may perform some tests or refer the couple to a specialist centre. The first step the specialist will take is to find out what the cause of the childlessness is. This is the process of diagnosis of both the male and female partners. Once a diagnosis has been made treatment can begin, if the couple want to and if the condition allows. In some cases, the couple know in advance what the problem is, as in the case of early menopause; cancer leading to the removal of the ovaries, womb or both; or infertility due to **chemotherapy** in males and females. Such couples may also present for treatment and some of the options described in later chapters of this book can provide a solution to their childlessness.

It is worth noting what the population size of the problem is. Estimates vary greatly, but there is some agreement that overall about 80–90% of couples who try to get pregnant do so after one year. This increases to 95% after two years (Cooke et al., 1981). However, if you consider the proportion of women not succeeding in getting pregnant when they are trying at any point, a prevalence rate of between 9% and 14% is indicated. The numbers failing to conceive appear to be increasing, which has an effect on service provision. Service provision is also affected by an increase in public awareness of the problem and by an increase in the treatment options available.

Infertility is the term used globally to describe a couple's failure to conceive after one year of regular sex without contraception. Infertility is therefore used throughout this book as a reference to involuntary childlessness. **Subfertility** is a term synonymous with infertility, but specifically referring to people who have been able to conceive at some point. **Sterility** is the term denoting a total inability to conceive. **Fecundity** is the term used for the individual's capacity to participate in the production of a child, and **fertility**, often used to mean the same as fecundity, actually refers to the bearing of children. In other words fecundity is really used as a biological concept, whereas fertility is used as a measure of live births, the **fertility index**. Infertility can be further subdivided into primary and secondary infertility. In **primary infertility** the couple have no history of a pregnancy; in **secondary infertility**, the inability to conceive occurs after one or more successful conceptions (though not necessarily leading to a live birth).

Of approximately 20% of infertile couples, about 1–2% are likely to be sterile. Infertility is a problem faced by both partners of a couple, though it is usually the woman who seeks help initially. Reasons for this may be that women have a more pressing need to have a baby or fear running out of (reproductive capacity) time, or because some men may find it difficult to face up to the fact that there may be something wrong with their fecundity. In fact the male–female percentages for the cause of infertility are about equally estimated at 40% for each. Some 20% of cases of infertility are not attributable to either the man or the woman, and this is termed **unexplained infertility**. Figure 3.1 illustrates the most common causes of infertility.

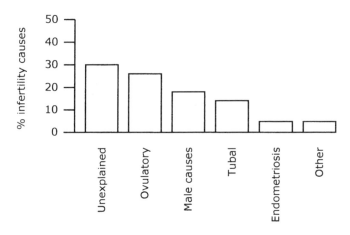

Figure 3.1   Causes of infertility

Fecundity is also age-related, and related to frequency of unprotected sex. In women the fecundity age declines with increasing years. For example, the optimum age of fecundity is about 24 years for women, with a decline seen at age 25–30, and a more serious drop in fecundity after the age of 30. For men, an optimum age in physical terms is not noted, although sperm quality tends to decline with age. Of course, with the changing socio-economic environment for women over the last decades, it is not surprising that many leave childbearing until later (van den Akker, 1994). Demographic variables, such as a high level of education, a high level of professionalism and a high family income, are social reasons for choosing to delay childbearing (van Balen et al., 1997b), and delayed childbearing is known to decrease fertility. The later age of marriage, or people forming lifetime partnerships, and the increase in **promiscuity** for men and women, also exposes more people to the risk of venereal diseases which are other possible causes of infertility. A recent report from the Public Health Laboratory Service has stated that sexually transmitted infections, such as chlamydia, are at their highest level in the UK since 1990 (*BMJ*, 2001), particularly so amongst women.

Unprotected sex four or five times a week increases fecundability. Despite frequency of sex and age of partners, the length of time a couple has been trying to conceive is associated with an increased likelihood of infertility. In other words, the longer you have been trying unsuccessfully, the less chance you have of conceiving.

The complexity of infertility is further demonstrated by the (not always understood) reasons why people want to have children. Hoffman and Hoffman (1973) developed the costs and benefit model, based on values, where children are seen as a source of social, psychological and economic costs and benefits to their parents. Although the model has been supported in some studies, Langdridge et al. (2000) used a different approach as they reasoned that the listing of reasons or values does not allow for relationships between them. They conducted a network analytic study to determine what reasons pregnant couples, in vitro fertilisation (IVF) and donor insemination (DI) patients gave for wanting to have a baby. Few differences were observed, apart from the result that DI couples ranked 'to make us a family' and 'to give a child a good home' higher than the pregnant couples, but not higher than the IVF couples. All three groups showed an emphasis on concepts such as the need to 'give love', 'receive love' and 'become a family' in the core network analyses. In general, research shows that happiness, well-being, identity, motherhood, continuity and social control are strong motivating factors for becoming a parent (Colpin et al., 1998).

Some couples may not be able to describe consciously what their reasons are; they may be too deep, or they may be there because of family, societal or other reasons. The main need for any couple wanting to have a baby is a sympathetic understanding of their problem and an appropriate approach to investigations leading to diagnosis and, if possible, treatment. The initial source of help sought by most infertile individuals is their GP. The GP needs to consider carefully when to refer a couple for advice or further investigations. If an individual is referred to a specialist, the GP should remain in touch with the patient(s) to reassure, explain and offer continued support. Many people will feel more at ease with their GP than with an unknown specialist, and specialists tend to communicate their findings to GPs in any case. Consequently, it is entirely reasonable and advisable to continue to approach one's GP about any further investigations or treatment, even if these are to be received from specialists.

One immediate effect accompanying this 'continuity of care' approach from the GP is that the isolation experienced will lessen, and psychological effects can be discussed. GPs can serve other purposes. They may be able to assist couples embarking on more unusual forms of treatment, to confirm support for their choice, and to help them with any doubts and uncertainties they may have. It is also important to know that anyone can terminate any treatment if the uncertainties become so great as to make the chosen treatment frightening or unattractive to the patient.

Once an initial diagnosis is made by the GP and confirmed by a specialist, the outcome may vary. It is possible that the specialist will tell the individual that there is no good physical reason why conception has not occurred. This may appear as both good and bad news. 'If there is no observable reason, then why has conception not happened?'; 'If there is no identified reason, does that mean we cannot get treatment?' These are possible questions that need answers. Second, it is possible that either a structural or functional reason for the infertility is found with a high degree of certainty, as the most likely cause of their failure to conceive. If this is the case, other emotions may rise to the surface. For example: 'Does it mean that I am incomplete or "not normal"?'; 'Why am I structurally or functionally incapable of conceiving?', and so on. Then there is the worry over treatments. 'Do treatments exist for my particular condition?' 'Are the treatments dangerous, painful, time-consuming, expensive?' 'And what are the success rates?'

Finally, a diagnosis of infertility may mean that conception or carrying a foetus is not possible. If this is the case, it is likely that people need to go through a **grieving** process. Following acknowl-edgement, acceptance or grieving, infertile couples may be able to turn their attention to other ways of having children and fulfilling the parenting function. These alternative options are discussed in later chapters. All that remains to be stated here is that fertility fulfils only one part of people's lives, albeit an important one for many – it is not the end, as many people may believe who reach this stage.

Although infertility is a private experience, it impacts on the provision of care, including economic factors and professional issues. These are constantly changing and the effects of infertility and the medical and technological developments to overcome them are constantly evolving. For example:

- Increased awareness of infertility and the options available to treat infertility results in an increase in demand for treatment (Page, 1988)
- Of all individuals undergoing treatment in the UK, 90% pay for it themselves because the NHS prioritises life-saving treatments over life-enhancing treatments (Gennaro et al., 1992; Kon, 1993)
- Health insurance normally provides a reduction in risk of financial loss when paying for health care services. However, infertility is generally regarded more as a social problem than a medical problem, with the result that insurance companies are reluctant to cover fertility services. This is partly based on a lack of societal agreement that these services should be included, and because accurate information about the appro-priate sequence of care and its cost-effectiveness has not been available (Tabbush and Gambone, 1998)
- Professional consideration of infertility as a specialist area has also been recognised (Fertility Nursing Group, 1990; HFEA, 1991) and is now undergoing change. The Fertility Nursing Group (1990) found that many nurses questioned in its survey felt inadequately prepared for their role. The changing needs of health care are now a prominent feature of the NHS. In order for professionals to respond to these changing needs, educa-tional programmes and resources must become more available, allowing staff to facilitate and implement treatments adequately for, amongst others, the infertile population's changing needs.

The private experience of infertility is therefore a recognised quality-of-life issue, now firmly rooted in the public domain. Infertility is dealt with by increased demand for better and more sophisticated treatment, services and economic factors, and more teaching for professionals and practitioners. Guidelines, laws, rules and regulations now enhance the public profile of infertility. The factual presentation of our internal systems, already discussed, will be addressed within the public domain in subsequent chapters.

The private experience of infertility has also been recognised as a social problem, and has been described as such as far back as documentation exists. Ironically, if society accepted womanhood without a prerequisite for childbearing the personal problem might not have become so great, as Miall's (1994) account of public infertility shows. For example, the Christian tradition sees children as a blessing from heaven and infertility as a curse or punishment. The Bible tells of the desire of Abraham and Sarah to have a child. They commissioned their servant Hagar to bear their child for them, although when Sarah herself later became pregnant, the servant and the baby had to make way for the new baby (the one with the full genetic link) (Genesis 16). Conceptions of motherhood and womanhood are based on the notion that motherhood is essential and is based in biological or genetic links.

Historical analyses of the cultural perception of infertility show some other interesting discourses. Marsh and Ronner (1996) examined the social problem of infertility and how it evolved into a medical problem in the early nineteenth century. Others describe the involvement of witchcraft in causing or healing infertility (Sade, 1994), the feminist theoretical and practical perspectives on infertility (Donchin, 1996), the religious and ethical perspectives (Spitz, 1996), and the environmental, evolutionary and natural forces perspectives of infertility. The literature is abundant and exciting, and each perspective lends itself to diverse yet meaningful ways of interpreting infertility in present-day contexts. However, the purpose of this chapter is to provide some insight into infertility as it is experienced today, and below I outline some common causes of infertility.

CAUSES OF INFERTILITY

There are many possible causes of infertility, and some may not be at all obvious or may even seem unlikely. However, clinical practice has shown that each of the causes shown in Table 3.1 may in itself or in combination with other causes be the basis of infertility. The general health of the woman is important for all normal physiological functioning. For example, we are all aware that smoking and excessive alcohol intake are detrimental to our health, with visible signs ranging from a more wrinkled, reddish-appearing skin to coughing and loss of appetite. Equally serious and perhaps less externally obvious are the effects of poor nutrition, which can cause biochemical imbalances or lead to anaemia, and **anorexia**, a psychological condition requiring intensive psychological/psychiatric treatment and which can in severe cases lead to **amenorrhoea**, the total cessation of menses, or even death. **Anxiety**, fear and other

Table 3.1   Common causes of infertility

Type	Female	Male	Female and Male
General/ *behavioural*	Dietary Anaemia Anxiety	Fatigue Smoking Alcohol Excess sex Fear Impotence	Relationship problems Sex problems Ignorance Low fertility index Immune incompatibility
Developmental/ *congenital*	Uterine absence or anomalies Hypoplasia Gonadal dysgenesis	Undescended testes Testicular germinal aplasia Hypospadias Klinefelter's syndrome	
Endocrine/ *hormonal*	Pituitary failure Thyroid disturbances Adrenal hyperplasia Ovarian failure Polycystic disease	Pituitary failure Thyroid disturbances Adrenal hyperplasia	
Genital *disease*	Pelvic inflammation Tuberculosis Tubal obstructions Endometriosis Myoma and polyps Fibroids Cervicitis Vaginitis Venereal disease	Mumps orchitis Venereal disease Prostatitis	
Cancers	Ovarian Cervical Uterine	Testicular	Any other treated cancers leading to infertility
Childhood *diseases*			Mumps

psychological effects can also influence somatic or physiological functioning. For example, anxiety has been shown to adversely affect blood pressure, hormonal and other biochemical/neuroendocrine functions. However, it is unlikely that **psychogenic** factors alone could cause infertility. Edelmann and Connelly (1986) assessed the likelihood of psychological factors leading to infertility and found no evidence to support this, although more research is needed in this area.

For the man, fatigue or exhaustion can have effects on the neuroendocrine system and, as with women, smoking, excessive drinking and fear will have similar effects. Impotence, the inability to perform sexually, can be brought about by a failure of the reflex system. However, in an otherwise healthy male it can occur for many reasons, both physical and psychological, and clearly poses a major obstacle in getting sperm transferred from the man into the woman. Excessive sex in the male has also been mentioned as a cause of infertility.

The last general category of both male and female causes of infertility relates to what may seem to many people to be obvious causes, yet there are many amongst us who do not relate simple behavioural factors to their lack of success in achieving a pregnancy. **Marital maladjustment** which, like any other psychological trauma, can be considered to be a major **life event**, or a deterioration in quality of life in one arena have both been demonstrated to have an influence on **somatic conditions**. Similarly, sex problems, which can range from erectile dysfunction to lack of desire, also have an influence on success or failure in conceiving. Ignorance, such as not knowing the optimum point in a woman's **menstrual cycle** for conception; **douching** or inappropriate cleaning of the vagina, and sperm leakage will all affect the chances of conception. The last of the general causes for infertility concerns a low fertility index, which relates to the formula expressing the ratio of one measurement to another; and **immunologic incompatibility**, which means that either the semen is rejected by the vaginal mucus, or vice versa, through an immune reaction against it.

Developmentally, as shown in Table 3.1, a number of structurally incomplete or abnormal conditions affecting the female are usually irreparable. In some of these cases, the woman may be born without the equipment needed to conceive or nurture a foetus. For example, some women may be born without a womb, or have a condition called **hypoplasia** which refers to the underdevelopment or defective formation of a tissue or part of an organ. **Uterine anomalies** (irregularities) and **gonadal dysgenesis** (a possible detrimental effect on later generations) are generally structural problems which cannot be corrected.

For the male, **undescended testes**, even if surgically corrected, often lead to infertility. Several other conditions can prevent males from being fertile. For example, **testicular germinal aplasia** refers to the defective development of the germinal tissues of the gonads; **hypospadias** is a **congenital** defect of the wall of the male urethra so that instead of the normal external orifice there is an opening on the underside of the penis; **Klinefelter's syndrome** is a condition where an individual is born with at least 2 X chromosomes which are nullified by the presence of a Y chromosome. The pattern may vary from XXY, XXXY, XXXYY to XXXXXY. Here the individual is physically male, but during puberty the testes fail to enlarge, facial hair is scanty and the pubic hair looks like that of a female. In some cases there is evidence of breast development. A person with Klinefelter's syndrome is infertile, and the more X chromosomes present, the greater the likelihood of mental retardation.

Some common endocrine causes of infertility for the man and woman include **pituitary, thyroid** and **adrenal** problems, including pituitary adenomas leading to the secretion of prolactin, thyroid dysfunction leading to an ovulatory disorder and adrenal disorders leading to **menorrhagia** and sexual dysfunction. In addition, other female endocrine problems may occur, such as **ovarian failure** to produce and/or release appropriate amounts of the relevant hormones, which will result in failure of the ovaries to function properly. In **polycystic disease** the problems of normal functioning are caused by many cysts. Genital diseases include **pelvic inflammatory disease (PID)**, an infection of the fallopian tubes which tends to involve the ovaries and peritoneum. PID can be acute or chronic. Acute PID is usually the result of an ascending infection and may be associated with the intrauterine device (IUD) used for contraception. The individual with acute PID may experience a period of much longer than usual bleeding followed by pelvic pain and irregular bleeding. Fever is common, as is tenderness of the vaginal area. In chronic PID the individual will experience pelvic pain which gets worse during periods, which tend to be irregular and heavy.

Tuberculosis (TB), although a rare disease in gynaecology, attacks the fallopian tubes and the endometrium and is likely to be transmitted sexually. Irregular menstruation and sometimes abdominal pain and infertility are associated with this rare gynaecological condition. **Tubal obstructions** can be the result of either abnormal early development or disease. If one fallopian tube is blocked but the other is open, there is still a 50/50 chance of conception. If both tubes are obstructed it doubles the likelihood of infertility. **Endometriosis** actually means a proliferation of endometrial (or uterus wall lining) tissue outside the uterine cavity. With 'internal' endometriosis the tissue develops in the **myometrium** substance; in 'external' endometriosis many areas, usually below the pelvis, can be affected (such as the ovary, bladder or rectum). No one knows how the process actually starts, but the stimulus of ovarian oestrogens has to be present for it to occur. The individual with endometriosis tends to be over 30 years old, not **parous** (that is, has not had children) and will have difficulty getting pregnant (although if pregnancy does occur, it tends to improve the condition). Pelvic pain is usually worst just before and during menstruation. **Myomas** are also obstructions to fertility, but are otherwise harmless tumours composed of muscle elements. These are non-carcinogenic (that is, not cancerous) and cause no further harm than preventing conception due to the obstructions they cause. **Polyps** are lumps of tissue which can be found in the uterine wall and are a result of incomplete removal of placental tissue following a pregnancy. These are usually diagnosed after heavy menstrual bleeding and can be removed using **dilation and curettage (D&C)**. **Fibroids** are circumscribed tumours with supporting fibrous tissue. They develop in the myometrium, and the location describes the type. Fibroids are the most common type of tumour found in women. They make the uterus bulky, and are associated with infertility. In fact, as fibroids are so common, the smaller ones are usually ignored, whereas the larger ones tend to be removed via ad hoc surgery or in the process of hysterectomy. **Cervicitis** is an inflammation of the uterus or cervix, and **vaginitis** is an inflammation of the vagina. Some types of vaginitis can lead to the formation of adhesions or false membranes between the vaginal walls.

Venereal diseases such as **gonorrhoea** are associated with sterility in both men and women. Other veneral diseases such as **syphilis** and **chlamydia** do not necessarily lead to infertility, though these diseases must be treated as soon as possible. Diseases such as gonorrhoea are not always easily detectable because the infection tends to be located around the cervical area and so awareness in the early stages may be difficult. Syphilis is a rare disease, but this can be detected externally as sores tend to grow around the vulva or penis, although infection can occur anywhere. As syphilis is extremely contagious the sores tend to spread rapidly all over the body a couple of months after contracting this disease. Transmission of the chlamydial bacterial organism is sexual, and in the woman the disease resides in the cervix, urethra and anorectum. Chlamydial infections are of several different types, but the one thing they have in common is that the disease organisms contain **deoxyribonucleic acid (DNA)** and **ribonucleic acid (RNA)**, and multiply like bacteria, although like viruses they can only multiply in host cells. **Mumps orchitis** is an acute infectious disease contracted in childhood. In the male, if mumps is contracted in post-pubertal years, complications such as orchitis can occur. Orchitis is an inflammation of the testes and is characterised by hypertrophy (enlargement), pain and a sensation of weight. **Prostatitis** is a term used for any inflammatory condition of the prostate gland.

Some of the above-mentioned diseases responsible for infertility are preventable. For example, the tubal damage caused by chlamydial infections could be reduced through effective population prevention programmes, including education and through changes in sexual behaviour. Prevention is better than treatment and is more economical in the distribution of health services and psychological distress. However, such disorders are still prolific in the population and show no signs of becoming less so.

CLINICAL CLASSIFICATIONS OF INFERTILITY

In clinical terms, other classifications of the causes of infertility used are shown in Table 3.2. These classifications are useful because they can be correlated with the testing procedures used in the evaluation and diagnosis of infertility.

The timing of sex seems an obvious factor to get right to achieve a pregnancy, yet it is surprising how many couples are not aware of this. The time just before and around **ovulation**, which usually occurs on day 14 from the start of the last menstrual period, is generally the most fertile period for conception in the woman. Ovulation is the term used to describe the ripening and release of the ovum from the vesticular ovarian **follicle** (see Chapter 1). Even when all other conditions are ideal, at least 40% of episodes of unprotected sex during the fertile period of the menstrual cycle do not result in conception. Frequency of sex is also relevant, because while infrequent sex can mean missing out on opportunities to conceive, too much sex can also lead to male infertility.

Table 3.2   Classifications of the causes of infertility

Classification	Includes:
Time	Timing of sex in the cycle
	Frequency of sex
Transport	Male: sex, tubal transport failure
	Female: sex, cervical, uterine or tubal transport failure
Semen	Sperm
	Other components of ejaculate
Ova	Growth and development of viable ova
	Ovulation
	Implantation
	Adequacy of corpus luteum
Incubator	Endometrial dysfunction
Other	Endocrine disorders
problems	Systemic diseases (for example, diabetes mellitus)
	Cancer
	Childhood diseases

Transportation problems are common in both men and women. These can be due to a variety of conditions ranging from congenital to viral or bacterial. The fallopian tubes in particular may be blocked or infected, or may simply not open sufficiently for ova to pass through. Similarly, the efficiency of transportation mechanisms of spermatozoa and semen are quite complicated. Both the sperm and the semen must pass through the reproductive duct system and must be appropriately ejaculated from the penis. Once ejaculated into the female, near the cervix, the woman's cervical mucus must be optimal for further transportation of the male ejaculate. Sometimes female mucus can be inadequate, with too much or too little progesterone or oestrogen. Immunologic incompatibilities between female mucus and male semen can also prevent the healthy transportation system.

Although little is known about the exact mechanisms transporting sperm towards the ovary while the ovum is moving simultaneously in the opposite direction, it is suspected that many causes of infertility can be found here. For example, with differentially dependent secretions, fine tubes and cell movements, it is inevitable that in some cases tubal dysfunction caused by infections, or endometriosis causing adhesions, may prevent effective transportation from taking place.

Semen is the term for the fecundating or fertilisation fluids of the male which contain the spermatozoa together with secretions of the prostate and seminal vesicles. In semen reflux, or the backward flow of semen, the semen is ejaculated into the bladder, which may be due to a congenital defect, or may be the result of a number of other causes including **prostatectomy**, a **posterior urethral stricture** or a **lumbar sympathectomy**. **Sperm** or **spermatozoa** are the mature male germ cells consisting of a disc-shaped head, a short middle body and an elongated motile tail or endpiece. The sperm must be motile (vigorous in movement, shape) in order to get to their destination.

Ova production and release during ovulation is dependent on a number of systems which must all function adequately in their own right. If hormone production is not as it should be, this will have an effect on ovulation. Follicles, too, must have the right environment in which to develop and mature. Ovulation itself must occur regularly, and the fertilised ovum must be supported. Adequate corpus luteum functioning is therefore also necessary.

The **incubator** is a name used for the endometrial lining of the womb, which, in normal conditions, is hormonally prepared in the post-ovulatory or premenstrual phase to carry a foetus to term. Appropriate adhesion to the endometrial wall, appropriate nourishment, and so on, is necessary for sustained growth. This is in part dependent on hormonal functioning. If the endometrium does not respond to endocrine stimulation of the ovary, pregnancy cannot occur. Adhesion of an embryo to the endometrium is also dependent in part on the quality of the lining of the womb, the endometrium. If the endometrium is severely affected by endometriosis, lesions and adhesions may prevent the embryo from implanting.

There can be many other reasons for, or problems resulting in, infertility and many of these are located elsewhere but impact equally severely on reproductive functioning. For example, **hypothyroidism** or severe **adrenocortical hyper- or hypodysfunction** may result in infertility. Usually the effect is on hormone secretions, thus affecting ovulation. Similarly, severe **diabetes** also appears to affect fertility, but exactly how this happens is not known.

PSYCHOLOGICAL AND SOCIAL EFFECTS OF INFERTILITY

Infertility, like many other reproductive system dysfunctions, has been investigated by professionals from many different disciplines. This is because infertility can affect many aspects of people's lives. For example, the psychological impact of infertility can be tremendous. This is not surprising because physical, social, occupational, personal and financial sacrifices have to be made. Monthly surges of optimism are followed by disappointment when menstruation starts again. Infertility has been described as a 'lifetime' crisis (Baluch, 1998). This crisis can also affect the professionals treating the infertile, since many couples expect an informed, involved and compassionate approach from the clinicians treating them. The clinicians may despair themselves, knowing they are doing what they can for the many couples they see, but feeling, as Mahlstedt (1985, p335) quotes, that 'I can't be all things to all people.' The effect of treating people in an area of medicine which changes rapidly is demanding upon the clinicians. New research and new techniques can improve the effectiveness of treatment. These advances also increase the need for developing skills and expertise in professionals, although the people needing the treatment are relatively constant. It is therefore not surprising that the 'people issue', the emotions and demands placed on infertile couples, is not always addressed as a priority in today's high-tech treatment clinics. This is an inadvertent result of training needs and the demands of clinical practice. However, the fact that the psychological functioning of the infertile individual is highly important is recognised, and efforts are constantly being made to address these as part of a holistic care approach.

A diagnosis of infertility can influence how the individual perceives his or her body and sexuality. Bodies can be seen as damaged or inadequate, and infertility may be seen as totally incompatible with good health. Scheduled sex and the clinician's discussion of an individual's often very private sex life may be seen as intrusive and may lead to an altered view of sexuality. Interest in sex can diminish dramatically as a result of this, and an inability to function or enjoy sex has also been reported (Mahlstedt, 1985).

There is a close link between psychological functioning and its influence on physiological functioning (and vice versa). Early research into the psychology of infertility has suggested that psychological factors can influence infertility directly (Pepperell et al., 1980), while other studies say the reverse is true. The most likely scenario is that a complex interaction between physiological and psychological functioning takes place. Cause and effect are difficult to assess, and these have not been established by infertility research to date. Instead an abundance of research has been carried out on the effects of infertility. For example, Menning has written several papers (1980; 1982) on the psychological impact of infertility, listing a number of common reactions to the condition which are also encountered when people grieve over the loss of a loved one. These observations have been confirmed by other research (for example, Robinson and Steward, 1996) and are considered normal reactions, although the intensity with which each can be experienced will vary. What matters most is that they are 'normal' reactions to bad news, and that, if each stage is worked through, the outcome will lead to a return to healthy psychological functioning. Menning's common psychological reactions to infertility are described briefly in Table 3.3.

Table 3.3   Common psychological reactions encountered in infertile individuals

Reaction	Description
Surprise	Shock and surprise are common reactions in the first stages of diagnosis, particularly if a couple has gone to great lengths to prevent pregnancy by using contraception
Disbelief/denial	The thought that 'this cannot happen to me' or there must be some mistake
Anger	When a couple gives control over their bodies to a clinician, the frustration and helplessness felt often turns to anger. Anger can also be expressed towards the partner, or towards other people who have unplanned pregnancies
Isolation	Isolation can manifest itself in two ways, either through thinking they are the only ones they know who are infertile, or by hiding their infertility from others
Guilt	Guilt is often assumed once infertility is diagnosed. If the partners used contraceptives, if they had previous sexual relationships, if they enjoy sex, if the woman had an abortion previously, or if a sexually transmitted disease was contracted – any of these factors may induce feelings of guilt
Grief	Once all hope for a pregnancy is abandoned, a necessary response is grieving, very much like when someone has died
Resolution	During this last stage, all or most previous emotions have been experienced and overcome. At this stage, a couple can live with the infertility although it will never be forgotten, or they may take some action

Other research has evaluated the impact of infertility using standardised psychological assessments, and depression and anxiety are commonly increased in many, though not all, of the populations studied (Harrison et al., 1984; Link and Darling, 1986; Freeman et al., 1987). These studies show how infertility can be experienced as a deeply stressful event which can have long-term effects on the individual's psychological health. It is important that this is recognised so that psychological health and coping are seen as part of the process, and that they can and should be addressed during treatment.

Not all individuals will experience either the diagnosis or treatment as stressful and not all will suffer psychologically (Connolly et al., 1993). Edelmann and Connolly (1998), in an excellent study in which participants kept weekly diaries, found little evidence of psychopathology and little evidence of distress or strain in relation to medical investigations, diagnosis and treatment. In fact, these researchers noted that some of the research which has been carried out has not distinguished between types of infertility experienced, types of treatment or even the stages of treatment their respondents were at during psychological assessments. Since different types of procedures which may have a different impact on the individual and the length of time of treatment (particularly if not successful) are important factors affecting an infertile individual's ability to remain optimistic, it is not surprising that individuals undergoing more lengthy procedures with less chance of successful conception will be more despondent than those who have just started a simple and relatively quick procedure with a high success rate. Nevertheless, it has given an overall picture of the scale of the problem, and that recognition in itself has great value.

Less intense psychological effects for specific groups of infertile individuals have been found by Connolly et al. (1993) in a **prospective study** of individuals at their initial visit to an infertility clinic and again nine months later. In this study, the psychological effects of different causes of infertility were considered separately. Overall, little psychological **maladjustment** was found. Men with male factor infertility showed higher anxiety and higher psychopathology than women with female factor infertility. However, these same men also tended to be (generally) **dispositionally** more anxious. In other words, it may not be a result of their infertility diagnosis but part of their psychological make-up. They also tended to be more likely to experience **marital maladjustment** (another good reason to be anxious).

In a recent study of infertile men in the UK, 84% reported stress associated with their infertility, and incidences of **depression** and **anxiety** were high. Men may find it difficult to discuss their infertility, and research has shown that if men do not seek professional support or 'social' support they tend to be more inclined towards anxiety (Band et al., 1998). These findings confirm those already described by Connolly et al. (1993), and men in this position could benefit from specific counselling. **Alexithymia** – the inability to communicate emotions – has also been found to be significantly higher in infertile males (though it is lower in infertile males compared to males with psychosomatic illness) (Conrad et al. 2001). It is likely that the depression resulting from the stress and loss of quality of life during infertility diagnosis and treatment is responsible for the increased alexithymia, rather than the infertility itself.

Other research has shown that good **attachment styles** between the partners in a couple are an advantage in terms of the likelihood of conception. Methods of coping with difficult situations also differ between people, and Mikulincer et al. (1998) have shown quite clearly that those with **coping styles** which are active, that is, they feel they can or are doing something about the situation (whether effective or not is immaterial), were more likely to adjust better to the stress of infertility. Levin et al. (1997) also reported that if task-oriented coping mechanisms are used by both partners, women report high marital satisfaction. High emotion-oriented coping by both partners, on the other hand, results in considerably more psychological distress for men.

Research into the effects on women's psychological health during initial infertility diagnosis uncovered similar effects. Domar et al. (1992) found significantly higher depression scores and double the prevalence of depression in infertile women compared to fertile women. They also found that the stage of infertility mattered, with those who had a short history of infertility being less severely depressed than those with a two- to three-year history of infertility. In their study, after about six years of infertility, depression scores were found to decrease again, presumably indicating that the women had come to terms with their infertility.

The **psychoanalytic** literature has also focused on infertility, although the angle taken tends to be different from mainstream psychology. In 1997, George Allison wrote about the revival of psychogenic causes of infertility. He referred to the fact that psychological factors can cause or contribute to the inability to conceive. He argued fervently against the idea that **psychogenic** causes were now regarded as obsolete and advocated their continued consideration. Allison backed his argument with three case studies of women unable or unwilling to conceive. The common underlying factors appearing in each case example were conscious and unconscious guilt and hostility towards 'a defective or deceased male sibling'. Although these writings may have little appeal to a large section of the population, the point psychoanalysts such as Allison are trying to get across is that infertility does present itself in psychoanalytic evaluation and treatment. It therefore needs to be part of the literature associated with infertility causes and treatments.

Saunders and Bruce (1997) studied the psychological mood state and physiological measures of stress in women during the months prior to and during conception. Their hypothesis was that stress levels would be lower during the conception months than during the months when no conception took place. Only 13 women were studied, but the assessment was detailed and prospective. They found that significantly more positive mood states were reported by these women during the conception cycles than during the non-conception cycles. They also reported fewer stresses during the conception cycle. Unfortunately, there was no clear relationship between the **adrenaline** and **cortisol** indicators of stress and the self-report measures across cycles. There could be numerous other reasons why women who did not conceive had a less positive mood. They could, for example, have experienced some **premenstrual symptoms** or **dysmenorrhoea**.

In short, the psychological effects of infertility can be non-existent, mild or severe. The recognition that infertility is not solely a medical condition is important. There is no doubt that in social, psychological and cultural terms, the inability to conceive can have an effect on one or both partners in a relationship.

FURTHER INFORMATION

Further information on infertility can be obtained from the organisations below.

Family Planning Association
2–12 Pentonville Road
London N1 9FP
Tel: 0207 837 5432
Fax: 0207 837 3042
www.fpa.org.uk

Foresight
28 The Paddock
Godalming
Surrey GU7 1XD
Tel: 01483 427839

HFEA
(Human Fertilisation and Embryology Authority)
Paxton House
30 Artillery Lane
London E1 7LS
Tel: 0207 377 5077
Fax: 0207 377 1871
www.hfea.gov.uk

National Endometriosis Society
Suite 50
Westminster Palace Gardens
1–7 Artillery Row
London SW1P 1RL
Tel: 0207 222 2776
Fax: 0207 222 2786

Klinefelter's Syndrome Club UK
Email: kscuk@klinefelter.org.uk

Daisy Network
[for premature menopause]
www.daisynetwork.org.uk

Miscarriage Association
c/o Clayton Hospital
Northgate
Wakefield
West Yorkshire WF1 3JS
Tel: 01924 200 799
Fax: 01924 298 834
www.btinternet.com/-miscarriage.association/

4   Diagnosis

HISTORY-TAKING AND EXAMINATION PRIOR TO DIAGNOSIS

Once there is enough doubt about the ability to conceive naturally, a couple is referred for history-taking before an accurate **diagnosis** can be made. Generally quite detailed histories are taken from both the man and the woman. Many areas are explored, and some or all may be relevant in reaching an accurate diagnosis. Sometimes aspects of history taken are addressed to rule possibilities out, as much as to rule them in. It is important that individuals are not daunted by this because the overall aim is to ensure as accurate a diagnosis as possible. Table 4.1 outlines some of the areas that may be considered in history-taking for the man and the woman. The table excludes areas explored in the physical diagnosis discussed later in this chapter.

Table 4.1   History-taking areas that may be addressed in a consultation

The woman	The man
Age	Age
Time spent trying to conceive	Time spent trying to conceive
Previous investigations	Previous investigations
The effect of childlessness on her life	The effect of childlessness on his life
Details of menstrual history	–
Details of reproductive history	Details of reproductive history
Sexual history	Sexual history
Contraceptive history	Contraceptive history
Medical history	Medical history
Social/occupational history	Social/occupational history
Psychological history	Psychological history
General health	General health
Abdominal/pelvic/cervix/uterus/adnexae and rectal examinations	Secondary sex characteristics/genitalia/penis/ cords/testicle examinations

There are great differences between the procedures faced by a woman and a man during the initial steps towards diagnosis. The first thing that will happen to a woman is that a thorough **history** is taken, followed by an examination and then subsequent tests for diagnosis. For the man, the reverse is usually the case. The first thing to happen will be the provision of a sperm sample from him, and this will be examined. Once the sample is declared abnormal, a full history will be taken and an examination will then be performed.

Age is important for the woman because the older she is the more difficult it will be for her to conceive. Time spent trying to conceive will obviously determine whether there is a problem. A 'problem' is defined as trying to conceive for about a year in women under the age of 35 and about two years in younger women. If a couple presents after trying for three months it is not considered long enough to warrant investigations because it is not against the odds of successful conception amongst the population. Previous investigations for infertility or other conditions need to be considered as much to rule out specific issues as to rule in their relevance. Another aspect relates to the desire for children. If the individuals are not too particular but are simply wondering why conception has not occurred within a given time period, it is probably not necessary to embark on invasive investigations followed by treatment. If, on the other hand, the individuals believe it to be a very important part of their life, further testing will be recommended.

Details of the woman's menstrual period are relevant, because she may have had spells of amenorrhoea or she may have started an **early menopause**. Bleeding irregularities or severe bleeding, on the other hand, could be indicative of endometriosis. Drugs can also affect menstrual functioning, and this is also considered in the history-taking examination. Table 4.2 outlines other areas explored at this stage.

Most of the above-mentioned procedures will be carried out by the GP, although some refer earlier than others. In general, though, the GP needs to make an assessment of the need to refer for specialist advice. One important consideration against immediate referral, if no obvious abnormalities are found in the history or initial examinations, is the fact that about 90% of couples will conceive within the first year of trying and as many as 95% within the first two years. It is because of the high percentages of conception after a period of one to two years that referral is usually delayed. Of course, there are reasonable exceptions to this rule, for example, in women over 35 it is considerate to refer earlier because age can work against the likelihood of conception. Similarly, when problems are suspected or clearly observed in the examination, speedy referral may be necessary. When an individual or couple is referred, either after a reasonable time period of trying to conceive without success or because problems are suspected, the referral is to a specialist – often a specialist clinic where a thorough diagnostic process will take place. These have a number of different names, for example, **assisted conception units** (ACUs), fertility clinics, or in vitro fertilisation (IVF) units.

Table 4.2   Other aspects of history that may be taken

Aspect	Description
Reproductive history	For example, previous abortions
Sexual history	For example, sexually transmitted diseases
Contraceptive history	For example, contraceptive pill use
Medical history	For example, diabetes, anorexia
Social/occupational history	For example, working in environments with toxic substances are all factors which could rule further diagnosis in or out
Psychological history	Tends to be taken to ensure the details are correct and to ensure that the pursuit of diagnosis does not pose a threat to the psychological well-being of the individuals concerned
General health	A history of the person's general health is also essential. A sedentary lifestyle, poor diet or obesity can all influence reproductive functioning and can be overcome through behavioural efforts

DIAGNOSIS OF INFERTILITY

A diagnosis of infertility means the identification of a disease or condition, indicated by the symptoms, the mechanical fault or the irregularity observed, resulting in infertility. There are several reasons why it is important to have a diagnostic evaluation of the individual's fertility status, once he or she has failed to conceive after about a year of trying. First, it is important to determine the exact cause of infertility. Second, the diagnosis will lead to a **prognosis** (a prognosis is simply a forecast of the course the disease may take), which may have psychological implications. Lastly, it allows a therapeutic option to be initiated.

Balasch (2000) has noted the change in the way the infertile person is investigated since the advances made in artificial reproductive technology (ART), from 'diagnostic work-up' towards a 'prognosis-oriented approach'. He urges for a re-evaluation of this approach, as 'incompletely evaluated patients can be recommended to proceed to ART following an accelerated and often incomplete work-up'. The traditional 'work-up' assessments outlined by the

American Fertility Society (1992) and the World Health Organization (Rowe et al., 1993) are not always adhered to (Glatstein et al., 1997, 1998; Helmerhorst et al., 1997) and this is increasingly becoming an issue of concern.

In 1996 the European Society for Human Reproduction and Endocrinology (ESHRE) (Capri Workshop) discussed some important factors in the assessment and diagnosis of infertility. For example, although it was noted that a cause of infertility is indicated by the result of any abnormal diagnostic test result, it is even more likely that an abnormal test result 'defines a cause of infertility only when treatment of this cause enhances fecundability in comparison with no treatment'. Thus the usefulness of the increase in offers of extended evaluations should be carefully evaluated as these offers may be neither essential nor cost-effective.

Diagnosis of infertility is undertaken by many specialist centres across the country. One in ten couples are unable to conceive within

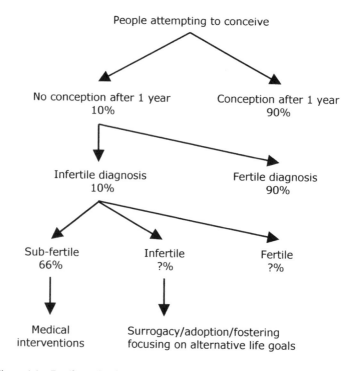

Figure 4.1   Fertile and infertile diagnoses by percentage

a year, and all of these can be investigated. A further 10% of the one in ten will be diagnosed as infertile. About two-thirds of them will in fact be subfertile, and they can be helped by some methods of assisted conception. (See Figure 4.1.)

CLINICAL/PHYSICAL DIAGNOSIS

For the woman, the simplest tests are **blood hormone levels** and **ovarian function** tests. Here a sample of blood can be taken and sent to a laboratory for analysis. Ovarian function can be determined in part from the hormone levels, from the occurrence of regular menstruation and from daily **basal body temperature (BBT)** measurements.

Subsequent analyses will determine if ova or oocytes are present. Without these pregnancy is not possible. Usually no menstruation occurs if no oocytes are present, but that does not mean that a woman cannot be amenorrheic with oocytes. If ova are present but no menstruation occurs it may be that there is no progesterone withdrawal, or if that is functioning well, that serum **follicle stimulating hormone (FSH)** levels are high (>40–100 mIU/mL). In this case, ovarian biopsy may not be necessary because the presence of more than 100 mIU/mL FSH suggests a certain lack of oocytes.

Ovulation means the release of a ripened oocyte from the ovarian follicle. This is relatively easily determined by BBT measurements. BBT is obtained by taking the temperature each morning before getting up from bed. Figure 4.2 shows a record of a typical BBT chart. Any normal thermometer will do, provided it is used properly. BBT is lower by about 0.3° to 0.6° just before ovulation and rises sharply as the result of the release of the hormone progesterone, indicating ovulation has taken place. Unfortunately, this is not accurate in all ovulating women, with some 10–20% of ovulating women not showing this biphasic pattern in BBT.

Once ovulation is determined it is time to concentrate on corpus luteum functioning. The corpus luteum is responsible for the production of oestrogen and progesterone. If this functioning is not adequate, establishing and maintaining a pregnancy are compromised. Inadequate corpus luteum functioning can show a short (less than eight days) luteal phase or a lack of progesterone production. The problems associated with inadequate corpus luteum functioning are more characteristic of secondary infertility (repeated abortion) than primary infertility (inability to conceive). Subsequent, more invasive testing may involve **laparoscopies** or **laparotomies**. These

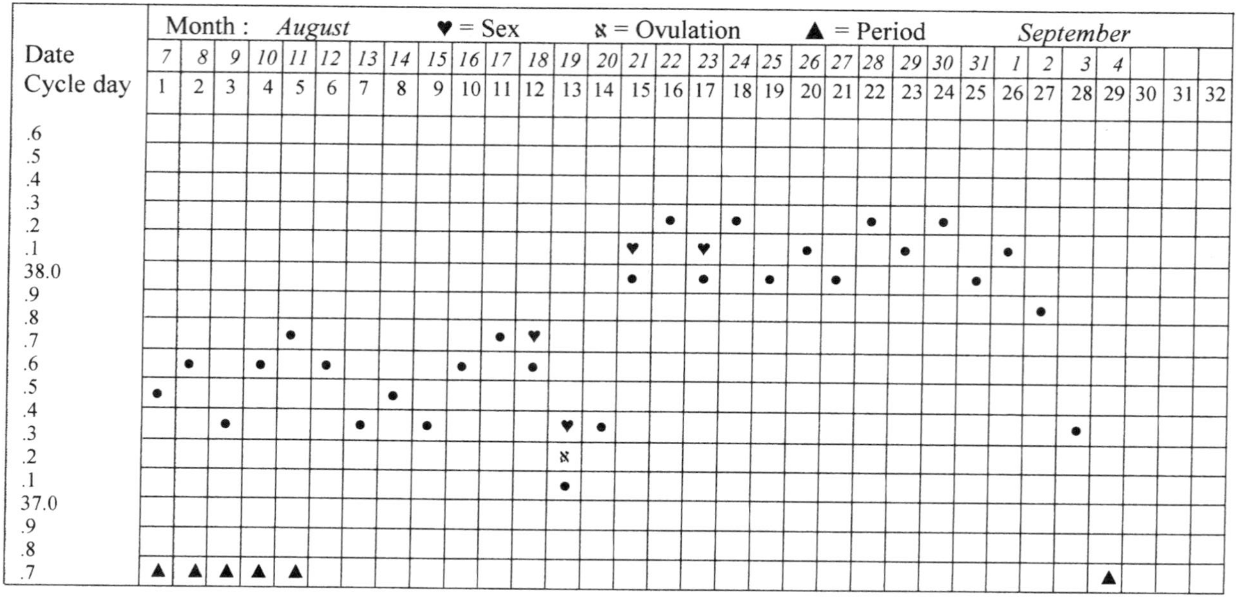

Figure 4.2 Basal body temperature chart

techniques involve the examination of the peritoneal cavity and its contents using a large laparoscope (a trocar with a light to examine the surface of abdominal organs and tissue) In laparotomies, an incision is made into the abdominal wall to allow further investigation of the chosen area.

For the man, the first step is usually the provision of a sperm sample. This can then be tested for mobility and motility, for adequacy of semen, or for chemical analyses of the seminal plasma. A sperm sample must be clean, and it must go straight from the penis into a sterile jar. This can be done through **masturbation** or **coitus interruptus** (coitus or sex where the man withdraws his penis from the vagina before ejaculation takes place). The man has to be sure that the entire contents of the ejaculate end up in the specimen jar. Usually more than one sample is needed to ensure that no mistake is made in the diagnostic process. The sample must reach the laboratory within about one hour of collection, and should not have been cooled or warmed.

In general, the more healthy sperm there are and the more active they are, the more likely it is that the man is fertile. Sperm counts below 10 million/mL or total sperm counts below 25 million per ejaculate are common in infertile men. Sperm counts between 5 and 60 million, or total sperm counts between 25 and 200 million are linked to a 50% pregnancy success rate, which goes up with increasing numbers or total counts of sperm per ejaculate.

Interestingly, between 3% and 5% of men have **autoimmunisation** with **circulating antibodies** to their own spermatozoa. **Autoagglutinating** antibodies tend to be present in cases where spermatozoa are clumping together, whereas **autoimmobilising** antibodies are present when motility of sperm is poor. Autoimmunisation itself is caused by an obstruction of the vas deferens, inflammatory prostatitis, orchitis, or through testicular biopsy. Nevertheless, in some 35% of cases no known cause can be identified. Of the two conditions, agglutinating antibodies give a better chance of pregnancy (about 50%) than immobilising antibodies.

A test carried out following sex, called the **post-coital test (PCT)**, is performed in the majority of clinics. Essentially the PCT allows for an assessment of sperm–mucus interaction, which relates to sperm-fertilising ability and is of value in the prediction of natural conception in couples experiencing less than three years of infertility. The usefulness of this test has been questioned because, whether the PCT is normal or abnormal, the treatment tends to be the same.

PSYCHOLOGICAL AND SOCIAL EFFECTS OF DIAGNOSIS

When a couple is trying to have a baby and nothing happens after a year, a sense of disquiet usually prevails. Many people believe they will never have a fulfilled life and feel incomplete without a baby. Others may see it as fate, or resign themselves to the fact that they have tried and failed, and focus on other aspects of their lives. Of those who are most disappointed, they may fear the investigations, the blame, or the resentment they may feel if one or the other of the couple is diagnosed as infertile. We know, however, that of the many infertile couples with a diagnosis (80%), at least 40% can be treated successfully. The first step therefore is to seek help together, to discuss the feelings and implications of a possible diagnosis in either party and to support each other during the process.

There are numerous emotions commonly experienced by infertile people. After the initial realisation they may feel surprise, denial, isolation and guilt, anger and depression. These reactions to infertility have been compared to grief reactions experienced by people who have lost a loved one. As with **bereavement**, appropriate acknowledgement of these reactions, sometimes with help from others such as a friend or counsellor, will result in appropriate **resolution** of the reactions. This need to resolve the feelings may not always be recognised by the individual or the professional, but it will be beneficial to all concerned if they are dealt with. Williams (1997) has given a psychoanalytic account of the 'profound need felt by the subjects for deeper understanding and compassion' with their plight. Many other professionals echo these observations from their clinical involvement or their research (for example, social work, Greenfield, 1997; medical anthropology, Gerrits, 1997; psychiatry, Rosenthal and Goldfarb, 1997).

The uncertainty of possible treatment outcomes can also leave a couple feeling isolated, anxious and depressed. It is essential that infertile couples receive adequate estimates of the success or failure of treatment, to keep them informed of progress, and to explain clearly why some options are available to them while others are not. A reasonably accurate estimate of the available options, if any, will help the couple to cope with future plans.

SEXUALITY DURING DIAGNOSIS

In addition to self-esteem and self-image, sexuality can also be affected by the diagnosis of infertility. Much has been written about women as childbearers, the role of women in society and the incompleteness of barren women. Similarly, men have traditionally regarded themselves as masculine only if they can affirm this status through the fathering of offspring. So for both men and women the consequences of infertility may stretch beyond the absence of the parenting function and affect their status as valid human beings, including as masculine or feminine sexual beings.

Having sex according to a prescribed schedule for diagnosis can remove the spontaneity and even the desirability of love making. **Post-coital** examinations and preoccupation with a BBT chart can make it difficult for both partners to perform. A general lack of desire, failure to obtain an erection and impotence are commonly documented during the diagnostic time period. Masters et al. (1992) acknowledged the procreative function of sexuality as one of the three types of sex (the other two types were recreational sex and relational sex). This procreational type of sex could be perceived as a continuum, from simply having sex without contraception to timing sex for the most optimum phase of the cycle. Seen within a continuum perspective, it may help the individual to realise that sex of this type is essential for reproduction and is only a part of the type of sex they think they have. It may then be possible to revert back to the recreational and relational perceptions of sex, in favour of the procreational type at a later stage in their attempts to conceive.

5   Regulation of Infertility Treatment

The UK Human Fertilisation and Embryology Authority (HFEA) plays an important role in monitoring good practice in all aspects of fertility and fertility care. It was set up in 1990 to safeguard and protect all individuals involved in licensed infertility treatment. It was the first such statutory body in the world and continues to have a great impact on clinical practice, particularly where new techniques are introduced. The HFEA also leads national debates on important ethical issues associated with any new reproductive technologies. Therefore, any clinic offering fertility treatment must have a special **licence** provided by the regulatory body, the HFEA. The HFEA provides all licensed clinics with their guidelines in their Code of Practice, which the clinics must all follow. The HFEA's guidelines for good practice include strict **monitoring** of staff, facilities, storage material, treatment, information given to patients, counselling, consent and costs. Failure to follow the guidelines can result in clinic investigations and a withdrawal of the licence. Failure to obtain a licence would be a breach of the law.

Reasons for the need for a regulatory body should be obvious. There are instances of **malpractice**, inadequate care and insufficient information provided to individuals opting for any kind of treatment. Those with fertility problems, as with any other condition, should expect the best possible care as the psychological, social and physiological implications of malpractice can have far-reaching effects.

Examples of the need for monitoring and regulation stipulated by the HFEA concern, for example, donor issues. The HFEA stipulates that all clinics using donor sperm must obtain the names and dates of birth of any donor to the HFEA. Other **non-identifying infor-mation** is also held on the register, so that when donor children reach the age of 18, they can access this **confidential register**. Access may be necessary to ensure they are not related to someone they wish to marry in the future. The benefits of donor anonymity are in fact currently being debated. Some argue that donor information should be kept confidential to ensure that people will continue to come forward to donate. Others argue for the need to disclose the donor's origins to any child, so that the child is aware of the truth of his or her conception, genetic origins and therefore lineage (but see Chapter 10 for more details on these issues).

Staff monitoring is also important. If a member of clinic staff does not wish to be involved in procedures they find objectionable for moral or other reasons, they are entitled not to part take in such procedures. Staff qualifications are also part of the regulations. At least one member of staff must be accredited/qualified to provide adequate counselling to clients as and when required. Adequate procedures must also be in place acknowledging and investigating complaints. In general, the expectation is that at least one identified senior member of staff should be available as a complaints officer. Facilities monitoring refers to issues of storage of gametes or embryos, as well as privacy for the provision of samples and for counselling purposes. This leads on to assessment of clients/patients and confidentiality issues. Consent for any procedure must first be obtained by the clinic from the patient concerned. Box 5.1 lists some of the types of consent which are needed before procedures can be implemented.

Box 5.1   Examples of consent required from patients

Consent related to:

- Investigations
- Treatment procedures
- Side-effects
- Risks involved
- Numbers of embryos to be transferred
- Fate of unused gametes
- Fate of any remaining embryos
- Genetic screening

No one is in a position to consent unless they have been adequately informed. Consequently information provision, without coercion, and timing and manner of information provision is also crucial. In assessing the appropriateness of treatment, clinics are bound by the regulations to consider the welfare of the child(ren) born as a result of the treatment. This is particularly important when multiple births are a possibility, where other members of the family may have different attitudes to children conceived through donation or artificial means, and where the child may want to know about his or her origins. Other possible concerns raised include issues of legal fatherhood of the child, and gestational/genetic motherhood in surrogacy cases. Most of these issues are addressed through each clinic's **ethics committee** or board.

The provision made for donors is also regulated by the HFEA. **Donors**, like **recipients**, must be well informed about the procedures, implications, emotional effects and risks involved in donating their gametes. It is important to remember that a man or woman undergoing fertility treatment can himself or herself become a donor, particularly if more gametes were retrieved or more embryos developed than were used in treatment. Here, too, genetic testing, numbers of donations possible, purposes for which their donated sperm or eggs may be used (research or treatment), and issues relating to anonymity need to be considered in detail. Other factors concern the realisation and appropriate counselling of individuals with regard to spare gametes or embryos, and what is to be done with these in the future. Individuals need to be in a clear frame of mind to decide what to do with these: whether donating them to others, allowing them to be used for research, keeping them stored for the legal period of time, or allowing them to perish.

If gametes or embryos are to be stored, the regulations specify that the highest standards should be maintained. Standards concern security, identification and storage review (time stored, contamination, ensuring they are actually there, and transfer). The HFEA's guidelines extend to conduct during research and record keeping.

Thus, the HFEA is the regulatory body for any treatment a patient may undergo for infertility. Once HFEA approval for a licence has been granted, the process between clinics is largely the same and follows a few logical steps, as laid down by the regulations:

- *Patients will be asked for a full **history**.* This is done to ensure that all relevant material is transferred from for example the GP, and any other is up to date, and that the clinician dealing with a patient's possible treatment has all the relevant information
- *Information about the clinic and about the possible treatments will be provided.* All clinics will provide a patient with written information about the clinic and about the treatment procedures

which are carried out in that clinic. The information provided will generally concentrate on the processes involved, but may also provide details of the staff. Costs, if the clinic or treatment opted for is private, will also be detailed in the clinic's information. The HFEA also provides patient information guidelines

- *Patients will be given **counselling** before treatment starts.* The recognition of counselling needs is also explicitly stated in several government publications (for example, DHSS, 1984, 1987). Counselling can be provided in different ways and is usually determined by the particular individual's needs. For example, one person may need a chance to talk with an impartial person about the long- or short-term implications of the chosen treatment. Another may need **supportive counselling** to help the person deal with the stress imposed by the treatment both in the clinic and at home, and others may require **therapeutic counselling**. The aim of all counselling is to benefit the individual's emotional and social (including family) needs and to offer support where necessary

- *Patients will be asked to provide consent for the treatment chosen.* This is usually written consent. **Consent** for treatment is necessary in all cases. However, the type of consent, and the numbers of consent forms a patient will need to sign will vary according to the clinic and the type of treatment received. In fact the correct term used here is **informed consent**, which means that the clinic will have informed the individual of exactly what the treatment involves and what the implications of the treatment are. Informed consent is a legal and ethical requirement, but this is still not always adequately delivered (Wear, 1999). If patients have not been informed, they cannot give informed consent. It is therefore important that prospective patients at a clinic make sure they are satisfied that they are well informed before consenting to the treatment.

There are numerous aspects to consenting for particular treatments which may not be at all clear at the start of the exciting possibility of becoming a parent. It is important to be aware of the implications of all aspects of consenting and treatments. For example, if donated sperm or donated eggs are to be used, neither the partner nor the patient have to consent to their use. This is because the donors will already have consented to their use. Other forms of consent refer to disclosure of information about treatment to other parties. For example, any clinic wishing to provide information about a patient's treatment to his or her GP, for example, cannot do so lawfully unless specific consent for all or part of the information is given by that patient.

If either the patient and/or his or her partner need to have sperm, eggs or embryos frozen and stored, their specific consent is needed. All separate male and female consents need to be matched so that the regulatory bodies have complete consent information on material belonging to all parties involved.

The next steps involve those specific to the chosen treatment. These will be discussed in some detail in the next chapter. There are as many different types of treatment as there are types of infertility, and the type of treatment will, of course, depend on the type of infertility.

FURTHER INFORMATION

Further information is available from the HFEA.

HFEA
(Human Fertilisation and Embryology Authority)
Paxton House
30 Artillery Lane
London E1 7LS
Tel: 0207 377 5077
Fax: 0207 377 1871
www.hfea.gov.uk

6 Treatments

In all assisted conception treatment for infertility, it is the clinic's responsibility to consider the welfare of any child who may be affected by the birth. Any diagnosis about the causes of a patient's infertility will already have been carried out (see previous chapters) before treatment can be considered. The diagnosis will have helped to determine the best treatment options for the condition. However, in addition to the availability of the results of tests to determine a diagnosis, additional tests may be carried out prior to treatment. These can include immunity to **German measles** in the woman, and **hepatitis B** in both the man and woman. **Preimplantation genetic diagnosis (PGD)** is also becoming more established in increasing numbers of infertility treatment centres. The technology used in PGD has evolved rapidly, and tests are now increasingly carried out to make accurate chromosomal and DNA investigations possible prior to implantation of the embryo (ESHRE PGD Consortium Steering Committee, 2000).

Treatment implies intervention, and in Artificial Reproductive Technology (ART) treatment the implication is that technology is involved. Technology aimed at better meeting human needs has developed at a rapid pace in recent decades (as will be discussed in later chapters). However, some form of improvement in meeting human needs has, of course, been going on for many years, from 5000 BC, when it was discovered that a better variety of corn could be produced if seeds from the best crops were sown, to the **cloning** of the first tadpole in 1952. Nevertheless, the skills involved in techniques used today require mind-boggling precision and have crossed boundaries previously thought impossible to cross. Despite this, the success of any treatment cannot be guaranteed. Instead, treatment today gives the *opportunity* for a successful outcome. Roughly 15–20% of assisted conception treatment cycles are successful and these percentages increase with each treatment cycle. It is therefore important to consider the fact that a less than 50% chance of successful conception is likely, depending on the technique used. Bearing these figures in mind, it is equally important to consider coping with disappointment – well over half the individuals undergoing treatment will not succeed.

Two further considerations are also necessary when making the decision to seek treatment. Most treatments are time-consuming and expensive. The individual embarking on treatment for assisted conception should be aware that time away from work is inevitable. For some this may mean loss of earnings, which may make meeting the costs of some treatments even more difficult. The average costs of treatments vary greatly depending on NHS availability of treatment and the amount of drugs needed.

Thus there are many factors that need to be taken into consideration before seeking treatment. Since different health regions purchase treatments differently, and private and NHS-funded treatment centres each provide their own statistics about the likely success rates for each treatment within their centre, it is important that individuals have an understanding of what these figures actually mean. Some of the points which need to be considered in any assessment of treatment effectiveness include patient selection, and outcomes.

When data are presented indicating success and failure rates overall or by specific treatment, it is worth finding out what type of patients were included in the results presented. Were these all patients seeking treatment, or only those who were most likely to benefit (for example, younger women) from a particular treatment? Was success based on **conception** or **live birth rates**? Were **spontaneous pregnancies** excluded from the results?

In terms of outcomes, it is necessary to consider not only the success and failure calculations of take-home baby rates but also the outcome costs to the individuals being treated. Were all aspects of care considered in the determination of successful or failed outcomes? Even if live birth rates are considered (a pretty solid-looking indicator of success) one needs to know if this included multiple births – not all will survive following delivery. Probably the best indicator is that which provides details on babies taken home. The reduction of stress or social disadvantage of infertility should also be incorporated into success or failure rates. A successful outcome, for example, would be a couple going home following resolution for their childlessness, particularly if this is weighed off against a couple undergoing multiple treatments over many years and adding to successful conception rates but not to take-home baby rates. The latter couple clearly are not a successful outcome case, whereas the former would be. Table 6.1 shows some figures for reproductive treatments in the UK in 1990.

Table 6.1   Reproductive treatment statistics for the UK, 1990

9,964 patients entered treatment
Each received an average of 1.16 treatment cycles

Treatment	Result
11,583 ovarian stimulations	15% failed to respond
9,829 egg collections	17% failed to fertilise
Of those who had eggs fertilised:	
8,195 embryo transfers were carried out	76% failed
2,004 clinical pregnancies	20% aborted
	3% ectopic pregnancies
	2% perinatal deaths
Live birth rates	74% single births
	22% twins
	4% triplets +

Source: Derived from HFEA (1992).

For those who decide to try treatment, the conditions which are treatable by specific techniques and the processes and procedures involved in each are described below, in addition to possible side-effects which have been reported for some treatments.

INTRAUTERINE INSEMINATION (IUI)/ARTIFICIAL INSEMINATION (AI)

Intrauterine insemination (IUI) or **artificial insemination (AI)** is a relatively simple procedure where fertilisation occurs inside the woman and not in a test tube, by inserting the sperm directly into the uterus. This procedure is the oldest type of treatment used when the following causes for infertility have been diagnosed:

- **anti-sperm antibodies**, a condition in which sperm will not penetrate the cervical mucus of the female partner. This condition is characterised by healthy sperm, but the male produces an immunoreaction to his own sperm
- tube defects in the woman, provided at least one of the woman's fallopian tubes is healthy (open to allow access)
- mild endometriosis
- unexplained infertility
- ovulatory disorders (provided they respond to fertility drugs).

There are different types of artificial insemination according to the sperm sample used. One is **artificial insemination by husband** (or partner) **(AIH)**, the other is **artificial insemination by donor (AID)** or **donor insemination (DI)**. In both cases the procedures and techniques are the same, but the sperm samples inserted into the womb are different.

If it is possible to use the husband's/partner's sperm then this will always be used, unless he has a genetic condition which contraindicates its use. In AIH, any resulting child will be genetically related to both partners. However, if the husband's or partner's sperm is not able to fertilise the egg, AID or donor sperm can be used. This means that the resulting child will be genetically related to the mother but not the father. If AIH is used, the partner will be asked to produce a fresh sperm sample, which will be prepared and inserted into the womb a few hours later.

AID or DI is usually chosen if there are problems with the man's sperm or if he carries an inherited disease which might be passed on to the couple's child. All donors will have been screened for some major diseases such as **human immunodeficiency virus (HIV)**, hepatitis and sexually transmitted diseases. For HIV in particular, sperm needs to be frozen and quarantined for at least six months. Once the donor sperm sample is certified healthy it is defrosted and placed into the woman's womb or cervix.

IUI can be carried out without stimulation of the woman's eggs. However, in most cases ovarian stimulation is now carried out in the woman to increase the chances of conception (see below). Figure 6.1 shows how the sperm is inserted into the uterus.

If the egg stimulation was successful and ovulation has taken place, the man needs to provide a sperm sample.

- The sperm sample will be prepared and placed either in the cervix or high in the uterus through a fine tube
- A period of 10 minutes' bed rest after IUI is recommended, as it has been shown to improve pregnancy rates in a recent **randomised controlled trial (RCT)** (Saleh et al., 2000).

The last step is to monitor the woman for signs of pregnancy, and tests are carried out to confirm a pregnancy. The success rates of IUI when **superovulation** (ovarian stimulation with drugs) is used are between 10% and 15%, but can reach 50% after several attempts in one year.

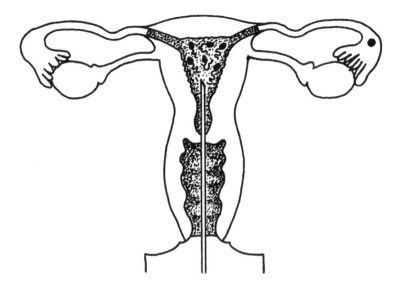

Figure 6.1   Insertion of sperm into the uterus (IUI)

Donor insemination is also used by individuals outside clinics. This type of donor insemination is known to be used by people who do not have a fertility problem, but who need a sperm sample to conceive for social reasons. It has, for example, been used by individuals within lesbian relationships and has been used in some cases of surrogacy. The procedure is far simpler than that described above because no stimulation with fertility drugs is required, and the sperm is inserted by the individual herself with a syringe or an instrument having a similar effect. The disadvantage of doing the insemination outside the conditions of a clinical environment is that there are risks associated with the use of unchecked sperm.

OVARIAN STIMULATION

Ovarian stimulation is very much a medically controlled form of treatment. Here, drugs will be given to the woman to stimulate several eggs to mature. Two drugs are administered: **GnRH agonists** and **gonadotropins**.

- GnRH agonists are administered to suppress all other hormonal activity. GnRH is administered by injection or through nasal sprays, usually for about two weeks. Then gonadotropins are given for a period of time, depending on the individual being treated and her individual response to these drugs. The woman may then take the GnRH for a further 10–14 days if necessary. Commonly used drugs are a GnRH drug called Nafarelin, which can be used as the nasal spray, and Zoladex, which is taken via subcutaneous injection

- Gonadotropins are given to stimulate the growth of follicles and to cause ovulation (the release of the mature ova). Normegon and Orgaful are examples of drugs used which emulate the action of hormones to promote the production of eggs.

Once these drugs have been given, the woman is monitored regularly using **ultrasound** techniques to measure the growth of the follicles, to tailor drug doses to that particular woman's needs, and to prevent serious side-effects. Monitoring is relatively discomfort-free by **transvaginal ultrasound** or by measuring **blood hormone levels**.

- Transvaginal ultrasound involves the insertion of a tube, illuminated at the end, which reflects the targeted object on a screen: in this case, the follicles. It is then possible to 'see' the growth of follicles. This may be done two or three times during a treatment cycle
- The measurement of blood hormone levels involves the taking of a small blood sample which is sent off for hormone assay analyses in a laboratory. The laboratory then returns numerical data back to the clinical team, indicating levels of specific hormone concentrations in the blood.

The most worrying aspect here is that no one has control over how the drugs will affect the woman and how many eggs will fertilise. If ovarian stimulation is used there is a fairly high chance that multiple embryos will develop, leading to multiple pregnancies. This cannot be predicted in IUI because the sperm is simply inserted into the woman and conception then follows its own course. If multiple follicles have ripened, they may all be fertilised. Alternatively, only one or two, or none, may fertilise. Multiple pregnancies carry a higher immediate risk for the woman and, depending on the number of babies, a higher risk of prematurity and associated problems. The condition referred to as ovarian hyperstimulation syndrome (OHSS) is very rare, but can be extremely dangerous and will be mentioned later in this chapter. On the positive side, the stimulated follicles should provide a better chance of in vivo (within the body) conception than if the woman's follicles were not artificially stimulated.

EGG COLLECTION

The procedure called **egg collection** means exactly what it says. Here eggs are manually removed from the woman's ovaries. In order to do this, drugs will be given to the woman to stimulate several eggs to mature. The same two drugs mentioned in the previous section, GnRH and gonadotropins, are administered. The procedure so far is exactly the same as that described in the previous section.

- GnRH agonists are administered to suppress all other hormonal activity
- Gonadotropins are then administered to stimulate the growth of follicles and to cause ovulation (the release of the mature ova)
- Once drug uptake is adequate, the woman is monitored regularly to measure the growth of the follicles, to tailor drug doses to that particular woman's needs and to prevent serious side-effects. Monitoring is again carried out by transvaginal ultrasound or by measuring blood hormone levels.

In IVF and other techniques where fertilisation occurs outside the body, eggs need to be extracted from the woman for fertilisation in a dish. The next step differs from the previous section on IUI, where eggs are stimulated. Egg collection is not carried out for the IUI procedure because fertilisation would occur in vivo, so there is no need in IUI to remove or collect the eggs. Unlike IUI, egg collection or harvesting usually starts about 32–36 hours after the last injection, and is probably the most invasive of the steps involved in IVF. Here the eggs are collected, usually under local anaesthetic, and the entire procedure lasts between 10 and 20 minutes.

The procedure follows some methods already familiar to the woman:

- Transvaginal ultrasound is used to guide the tube actually collecting the eggs
- The eggs are collected through a small tube or catheter, by placing it next to the ultrasound through the vagina. Alterna-

tively, the tube can also be inserted laparoscopically, through the abdominal wall. When laparoscopic egg collection is performed, a general anaesthetic is necessary. Once the eggs are visible and the tube is in position adjacent to the eggs, suction from the tube collects the eggs and the suction tube carries them directly to the dish in the embryologist's chamber (usually next to the treatment room). During transvaginal egg collection, when a local anaesthetic is used the woman can usually see the video screen of the tube and disc where an amplified picture of the egg collection is visible

- Anywhere between 1 and 40 eggs can be collected at any one time. If many eggs are collected, the best-quality eggs can be selected for fertilisation. The greater the number of eggs collected, the greater the supply of embryos for use in repeated treatment attempts.

IN VITRO FERTILISATION (IVF)

In vitro fertilisation, or **IVF**, is often called the 'test-tube' treatment. Here the fertilisation of an ovum occurs outside the body. In IVF treatment, the eggs are collected from the woman's ovaries (discussed in the last section), and the man's sperm is mixed with the eggs in a test tube (see Figure 6.2). The sperm may fertilise one or more eggs, which are left to culture for about a day to ensure normal development. If this part of the procedure is successful, the resulting fertilised embryos are transferred into the woman's womb, as diagrammatically shown in Figure 6.3. Usually, no more than three embryos will be transferred at any time. Any remaining fertilised embryos are usually frozen. There is much current debate about whether transferring three embryos is too many, but this will be discussed further in Chapter 11. There is then a waiting time to see if one or more embryos will implant in the lining of the womb. As in normal conception, the implantation will be the beginning of a successful pregnancy. The technique was originally developed to treat couples whose main cause of infertility was tubal damage, but nowadays it is used to treat the problems listed below, and even to treat unexplained fertility.

- Endometriosis
- Blocked fallopian tubes
- Cervical mucus problems
- Male factor infertility

- Older women whose eggs will not fertilise, or who have had ovarian disease or surgery (donated eggs can be used).

Although IVF is probably the most widely used treatment for infertility around the world, its success rates need to be taken into account. After one cycle of treatment, success rates of conception are about 25%, with a lesser chance of delivery. The take-home baby rate is about 15% for each cycle of treatment. Babies born through IVF are often referred to as **'test-tube babies'**, and many people will remember the pioneering achievements of Edwards and Steptoe in 1978 when the first ever test-tube baby, Louise Brown, was born through this method. Today, IVF is carried out by many clinics throughout the UK, and each needs a special licence from the HFEA licensing authority to ensure good practice following accepted procedures.

The IVF procedure follows several steps, and each takes a considerable amount of time because the individual and specialists, the obstetric team and the embryologist, have to work to the woman's menstrual cycle.

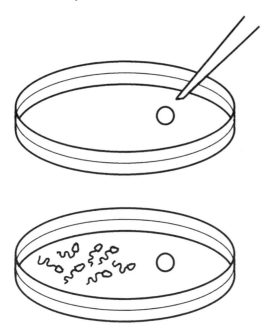

Figure 6.2   Test-tube mixing of egg and sperm

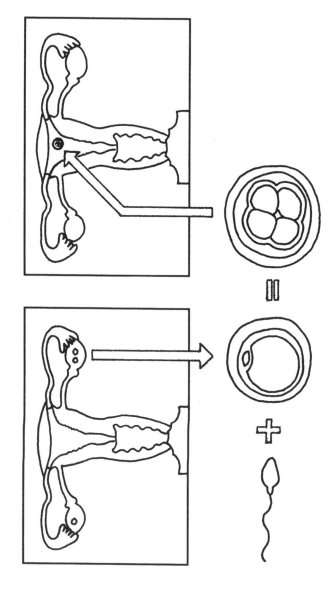

Figure 6.3   Embryo transfer to uterus (IVF)

Initially drugs will be given to the woman to stimulate several eggs to mature. The procedure is identical to that described in the earlier section on ovarian stimulation.

- Drugs are administered to stimulate several eggs to mature (see section on ovarian stimulation)
- The clinical team then is ready for the egg-collection procedure
- Once drug uptake is adequate and the follicles are growing, the woman is ready to have her eggs removed, collected or harvested (see section on egg collection).

If the egg collection is successful, the quality of the eggs will be determined and, if all is well, a sperm sample will be asked for on the same day as the eggs were collected.

- Here the man needs to ejaculate into a jar, and this sample too will be analysed.

All is now ready for fertilisation in vitro (outside the body). **Fertilisation** is the term used when one or more sperm has successfully penetrated the egg, and cell division has started.

- The eggs and sperm will be prepared for fertilisation. They will be inserted together into a petri dish, a small glass dish with a lid, where will be cultured overnight. 'Cultured' means they are allowed to grow
- The next day, the cultured sample will be analysed microscopically and the number and quality of fertilised eggs will be counted.

A couple of days after fertilisation in the tube (dish), the embryo will be transferred into the uterus of the woman. This again involves some steps the woman is already familiar with.

- No more than three embryos will be transferred at a time, but this depends on the clinic and the country where the procedure is carried out
- The embryo transfer is carried out transvaginally (through the vagina)
- The embryos are placed past the cervix into the womb

- Any spare embryos will usually be frozen for later use if implantation fails. Alternatively, they may be shared by another recipient patient of IVF, or remain stored for future use.

The last step is to monitor the woman for signs of pregnancy, and tests are carried out to confirm this.

Until recently only fresh eggs were used in IVF treatment, although eggs have been stored in freezers for several years and successfully thawed. UK clinics were not allowed to use these frozen eggs (subsequently thawed) in treatment until a change in the law early in the new millennium. A report by an independently commissioned individual has highlighted that the technique of using frozen eggs in IVF, although not without risks, has encouraging results. The HFEA consequently lifted the ban on their use (Wise, 2000).

OOCYTE DONATION

Oocyte donation has been a possible solution for the treatment of women who cannot provide their own ova. As in sperm donation, another person is needed to provide the gametes. However, unlike sperm donation, an ovum donor is required to undergo invasive medical treatment involving ovarian stimulation and the transvaginal retrieval of mature oocytes under local anaesthesia. This technique has only been a possible treatment option since the development of IVF, as it requires the donated ova with sperm (once an embryo is established) to be transferred to the recipient woman. This is called **embryo transfer**, or **ET**.

This option is appropriate if the woman has ovarian problems, particularly:

- primary ovarian failure
- premature ovarian failure
- women with normal ovarian function but who have had recurrent IVF failures
- women aged 43 years or over, because they tend to have a low success rate with their own oocytes.

The procedure following the harvesting of ova from the donor is the same as for IVF and ET (see previous section on IVF; also p. 61).

Donors can either be known or anonymous. **Known donors** tend to be female relatives or good friends of the woman with fertility problems. **Anonymous donors** are unknown to the recipient and are either paid a small amount of money (not for their contribution, but for reasonable expenses incurred) or they are donors who share their spare eggs in cases of '**egg-sharing**' practices. Egg sharing is a procedure encouraged in the UK since 1996. Here no additional risks are incurred, as the patient is already undergoing treatment for egg collection. Using this system of donation, donors (IVF patients) share their oocytes equally with a matched anonymous recipient. The recipient tends to pay for the cost of egg collection. Thus medical intervention is undergone by one patient while the other bears the financial cost of the procedure. There are some psychological implications of egg sharing which require consideration at an individual level, as well as at a societal level. It is possible, for example, that a donor IVF patient fails to conceive and the recipient does conceive. It may be tremendously difficult for the IVF patient donating her eggs to another patient to come to know that the baby she so desperately wanted has been successfully implanted in another woman. It will be the other woman who will take the baby home and care for it as her own. This has to be borne in mind when taking part in an egg-sharing scheme.

INTRACYTOPLASMIC SPERM INJECTION (ICSI)

Intracytoplasmic sperm injection (ICSI) is the newest technique available, and is considered revolutionary because it offers a viable solution to many cases of male infertility. It involves sperm **micromanipulation** performed in the laboratory. The success rates are equal to or better than IVF. ICSI has also been used to assist conception in women over 40 with existing ovarian function, but who may have a reduced reproductive potential because of their age. However, although some centres have shown that this technique – using supernumeracy embryos that are **cryopreserved** and transferred in subsequent cycles – can improve pregnancy rates, miscarriage rates are very high (for example, Nikolettos et al., 2000).

The technique is useful for:

- severe sperm defects, for example, globozoospermia, immotile spermatozoa, epididymal and testicular spermatozoa, elongated and round spermatids. It has also been used in preadolescent boys subject to chemo- and radiotherapy to have their gametes (secondary spermatocytes, spermatids and/or spermatozoa) cytopreserved for future use before treatment
- sperm counts of less than 5 million per millilitre

Aspiration
of the sperm

Injection of the
sperm cell into
the oocyte

Confirmation
of fertilisation

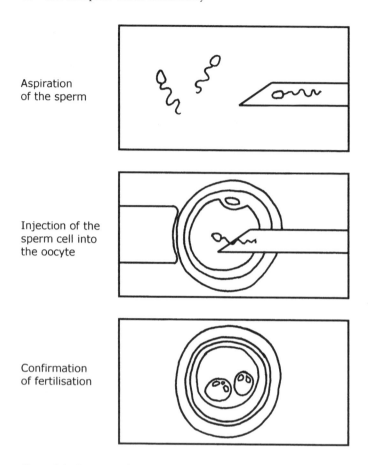

Figure 6.4   Intracytoplasmic sperm injection (ICSI)

- no sperm at all, because of blockage or other testicular disorders.

In this technique the sperm sample is obtained from the man through ejaculation or aspiration of semen from the epididymis (testicle). One single sperm is then injected into the cytoplasm of a single mature egg or oocyte using a microinjection pipette or thin glass needle (see Figure 6.4), retrieved earlier, as described in the section on egg collection. The resulting fertilised embryo is then transferred into the woman.

The ICSI procedure is extremely detailed and requires the manipulation of minute cells, requiring a high amount of precision. In addition, the woman's and man's part in this can be arduous. The procedures are briefly outlined below, as some of the precursor techniques involved have already been described in previous sections.

- As with many other treatments, ovarian stimulation is the first step
- Once drug uptake is confirmed, the woman is monitored regularly to measure the growth of the follicles through transvaginal ultrasound and measurement of hormone levels
- The next step involves egg collection from the woman into the embryologist's dish
- If the previous procedures were successful, a sperm sample will be asked for from the man the same day as the eggs were collected.

In the case of male infertility, it is possible that one of two alternative methods of sperm extraction is used, if ejaculation is contraindicated.

- The **microsurgical epididymal sperm aspiration (MESA)** technique involves inserting a fine needle into the epididymis and extracting a small sample of semen. This can be done under local anaesthectic, and takes about ten minutes
- Alternatively, **testicular sperm extraction (TESE)** is used. This technique is similar to MESA, except that a small amount of testicular tissue is removed and the sperm cells are extracted from that tissue.

All is now ready for fertilisation, which is carried out using microscopic manipulation of the gametes.

- Using ICSI, the egg is held at the end of a fine suction pipette so that it cannot slip away. Only one single sperm cell is inserted into a syringe with an incredibly fine needle. The needle with the sperm cell is injected directly into the egg. Following successful injection of the sperm cell into the egg, the egg will be put into a petri dish and allowed to develop
- The next day, the cultured sample will be microscopically analysed, and fertilisation will be confirmed.

A variation on the ICSI is a technique called **subzonal insemination (SUZI)**. Here an attempt is made to fertilise an egg by injecting not one but several sperm into the space between the egg cell's membrane and the **zona pellucida** (the outer coating surrounding the egg).

A couple of days after fertilisation in the tube (dish), the embryo will be transferred to the uterus of the woman. This again involves some steps the woman is already familiar with.

- No more than three embryos will be transferred at a time
- The embryo transfer is carried out transvaginally (through the vagina)
- The embryos are placed past the cervix into the womb
- Any spare embryos will usually be frozen for later use, if implantation fails.

The last step is to monitor and test the woman to see if pregnancy has occurred.

GAMETE INTRAFALLOPIAN TRANSFER (GIFT)

Gamete intrafallopian transfer, or **GIFT**, requires more invasive procedures than those used in IVF embryo transfer, as shown in Figure 6.5. Here the woman needs to have healthy tubes because that is where the eggs are collected from, and that is also where, as in nature and unlike in IVF, fertilisation will take place. Pregnancy rates for GIFT are reported as somewhat higher than for IVF, reaching approximately 36% per treatment cycle. The average take-home baby rate is also higher, at 26%. However, the range of fertilisation and conception rates will vary by clinic for all techniques. GIFT is currently used to treat several infertility conditions, including:

- mild endometriosis
- unexplained infertility.

For GIFT, much of the preparation or treatment of the woman is the same as that described for IVF, but in GIFT, fertilisation does not take place in a test tube.

With GIFT, as for IVF:

- ovarian stimulation will be carried out

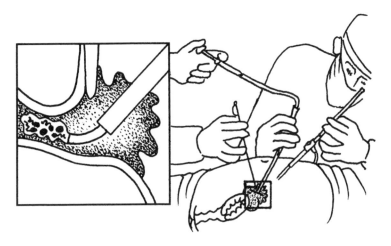

Figure 6.5   Gamete intrafallopian transfer (GIFT)

- egg collection will then be performed, although this tends to be done with a laparoscope requiring a general anaesthetic
- the provision of a sperm sample is then required.

The sperm sample will also be analysed for quality and health. This sample will be held in the operating theatre, ready for mixing with the woman's eggs. The eggs will also be examined for quality, and usually no more than three of the best ones will be selected for use in GIFT. Finally, the two samples, the sperm and the eggs, will be mixed together. The eggs and sperm, now mixed together, will be immediately placed back into the woman's fallopian tube, using the laparoscope to guide and the suction tube to reinsert them.

ZYGOTE INTRAFALLOPIAN TRANSFER (ZIFT)

Zygote intrafallopian transfer (ZIFT) is a technique which lies somewhere in between IVF and GIFT. In ZIFT, the actual fertilisation of the egg is carried out and confirmed in the laboratory. The **zygote** is then transferred to the fallopian tube. Unlike in GIFT, therefore, one already knows fertilisation has taken place, because this was confirmed in the laboratory before transfer to the fallopian tube. However, unlike IVF, the zygote does not get placed in the uterus, but in the fallopian tube. The technique is demonstrated in Figure 6.6.

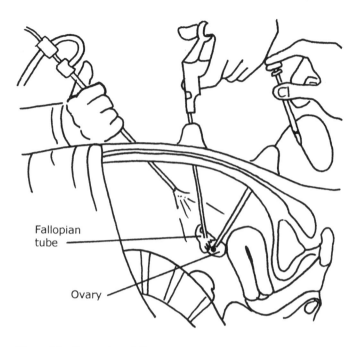

Fallopian
tube

Ovary

Figure 6.6   Zygote intrafallopian transfer (ZIFT)

ASSISTED HATCHING – EMBRYO MICROMANIPULATION

Assisted hatching is a technique which, as the term implies, involves the artificial (or assisted) creation of an opening in the outer covering of the zona pellucida of the embryo. It is a technique used to help the normal growing embryo to emerge from the covering in order to implant properly in the uterus.

SUMMARY OF INFERTILITY TREATMENTS

The knowledge of artificial reproductive techniques, the skill involved and the enormous sacrifices the individuals undergoing the treatment must accept have reached phenomenal levels. The results of such treatments allow a great number of previously childless couples to become parents. This, for most people undergoing these options, is one of the most important goals in their lives.

However, with treatment successes there are an equal number who need repeated treatments, and many more who will not be sucessful. All infertile individuals opting for treatment are informed of the success and failure rates and are expected to be both optimistic (to take this laborious route in the first place) and realistic (to understand and accept that most treatment cycles result in failure to achieve a pregnancy). Even if a pregnancy is confirmed, **miscarriage** is common, as are complications resulting from multiple pregnancies. Last but not least, a great deal of people opting for ART will at some point have to give up altogether. There are many reasons for giving up treatment, some of which are given in Box 6.1.

Box 6.1   Reasons for giving up treatment

- No embryos left
- The woman is too old
- Psychologically contraindicated to continue treatment
- Physically contraindicated to continue treatment
- No donor gametes available
- NHS limit of three free cycles fulfilled
- Financial reasons

Everyone involved in ART is motivated by the same aim: to achieve treatment success. The more sophisticated the technique, the more likely that success rates will improve. This implies that the more we intervene, the further we can push the barriers of what constitutes success. How success is measured depends on your outlook, and this aspect is to some extent covered again in Chapters 11 and 13. Of more immediate concern are the physical side-effects of treatment, which I turn to now, followed by a discussion of the psychological and social effects of the treatments discussed thus far.

PHYSICAL SIDE-EFFECTS

Side-effects are not unexpected with increasingly sophisticated procedures necessary to execute some of the reproductive interventions currently available. Most people will not suffer too many side-effects; others will perceive mild symptoms as severe, or severe symptoms as acceptable; yet others will suffer considerable discomfort. There is huge variation in how physical side-effects are perceived and in how they are subsequently interpreted or remembered. Weaver et al. (1997) report that some infertility treatments are often physically and psychologically painful. As with labour pain, it is often said that 'one forgets', particularly if the outcome is positive. However, there are some side-effects which need to be noted which occur in a proportion of people treated. The side-effects described briefly below are unequivocal side-effects resulting directly from the procedures used to improve quality of life.

- *Pain* is often experienced when egg collection takes place. However, there is no need for undue suffering, and painkillers can be given for this procedure
- *Bleeding* is common after tubal extraction of eggs, from the vagina, bladder or urethra. This is normal and not dangerous unless the bleeding is heavy, when the individual should seek advice. Cramping may accompany the bleeding, similar to the experience of dysmenorrhoea
- *The side-effects of drugs* can be numerous, and most side-effects disappear and usually are not serious. Some of the reported unpleasant but mild side-effects include hot flushes, depression, irritability, headaches and restlessness. Over-response to the drugs where too many eggs develop can occur, and in some cases cysts may appear on the ovaries or fluid may collect in the abdominal cavity. If this happens it can be controlled, although it is likely that the treatment cycle with a relatively unpleasant reaction to drugs will have to be abandoned – known as an '**abandoned cycle**'. This means that if the patient wishes to restart the treatment, she will have to go through this procedure again
- The condition called **ovarian hyperstimulation syndrome (OHSS)** has been known to occur in a few cases, and is the most serious complication of fertility treatment. It is extremely rare that the reaction to ovarian stimulation is this bad, but it is an effect that the individual should be aware of. Here a very large number of eggs develop in the ovaries, leading the ovaries to swell. The symptoms of this condition include shortness of breath, abdominal pain and swelling, nausea and vomiting, weakness and fainting. Anyone with this condition needs to be hospitalised immediately. Kol and Itskovitz-Eldor (2000) report that the threat of OHSS is preventable if ovulation is triggered using gonadotropin-releasing hormone GnRH agonists instead of human chorionic gonadotropin (HCG). However, contro-versy over the effective eradication of OHSS remains

- Side-effects can also occur with a **general anaesthetic**. Some people have no adverse reactions to anaesthetic, but many do
- **Multiple pregnancies** can be considered amongst the side-effects, although strictly speaking they are not side-effects. In multiple pregnancies the risks to the mother and foetuses are higher. Higher rates of pregnancy loss or miscarriage, and lower birth-weight babies tend to be common in multiple pregnancies. (Chapter 11, on ethical issues, discusses some of the problems of multiple pregnancies, including the issue of **foetal reduction**)
- The incidence of **congenital** malformations following treatments has been studied by Ericson and Kallen (2001). They carried out a population-based study of infants born after IVF and reported that in general, when confounders were taken into account, no excess of congenital malformations registered in the Medical Birth Registry in Sweden were observed. However, for neural tube defects and some other conditions a threefold excess risk was observed (some only following the use of specific techniques).

PSYCHOLOGICAL AND SOCIAL EFFECTS OF TREATMENT

Some of the most common medical treatments for infertility have been described in the previous sections. The effects of any treatment which manipulates the organism can be manyfold, and clearly if the treatment is successful the psychological effects will be different than if treatment is not successful. Few studies have examined the cause and effect relationships between psychological stress reactions and reproductive outcome. However, one rare study by Milad et al. (1998) hypothesised that since we know that psychological 'stress' reactions affect physical stress indicators such as the secretion of cortisol, prolactin and progesterone, it is not unreasonable to assume that psychological factors may directly affect pregnancy outcome in IVF-treated patients. Surprisingly, perhaps, these authors found no relationship at all between amount of stress and hormone concentrations or pregnancy outcome. In fact stress was reported as high in all participants – those who did have a successful pregnancy outcome (n = 22) *and* those who did not (n = 18). In general, treatment for infertility, though physically and mentally demanding, has rewards beyond the traumas of the treatment if the outcome is successful.

Many other research studies have carried out psychological assessments on people treated unsuccessfully with IVF, and the results generally show increases in depression and anxiety. This is not surprising considering the feelings expressed after initial diagnosis of infertility. If an infertility diagnosis is hard to digest, then unsuccessful treatment is equally likely to be hard to accept. However, as with diagnosis of infertility, many factors are relevant and influence how treatment affects a person, as each person's predisposition to emotional vulnerability will be different.

Psychological research has struggled with the same complexities here as those described in Chapter 4. Elevated depression, particularly amongst the female partners, is commonly observed (Mahlstedt et al., 1987; Baram et al., 1988), as is depression within normal limits in other studies (Freeman et al., 1987) or depression in both partners (Leiblum et al., 1987). Two factors are important here: one is the need to find out at what stage people are most affected by unsuccessful treatment, that is, immediately after treatment or much later; another is who is most at risk for developing psychological problems following treatment failure.

Newton et al. (1990) examined people referred for IVF treatment before the procedure, and again three weeks after their first IVF attempt. More anxiety pre-treatment was observed in women than men, but after treatment failure both men and women showed increased levels of anxiety and depression, although depression levels in the men were considerably lower than in the women. Again, these researchers found that if anxiety levels were high pre-treatment, they were more likely to be high, and usually higher, at post-treatment failure. Exactly the same was true for pre- and post-treatment failure depression scores. As with all these studies, it is important to point out that significant depression or **clinical depression** or anxiety is only apparent in a relatively small proportion of people studied. That proportion is clearly more vulnerable emotionally, and it is these people who would benefit most from some form of psychological help.

Studies such as these also confirm that men and women appear to cope differently with infertility. Women, on some marital and life adjustment scales, tend to be more openly expressive of feelings and more likely to seek emotional support than men, who tend to evaluate achievement orientations consistently more highly than women (Newton et al., 1990). Clearly, what is important is that men and women who are vulnerable to depression or anxiety prior to and following failed treatment would benefit from anxiety management training, in order to better manage the stress of treatment procedures and to help them to cope with treatment failure. Improved psychological preparation for treatment appears to be called for. Psychological distress as a result of **repeated failure** may be even higher than is reported for first time failure of treatment, and this needs further consideration in the future. Boivin et al.'s (1998) study failed to show differences between spouses in a prospective study assessing daily mood during one cycle of ICSI or IVF, but found the most important determinant of mood change was the uncertainty of the treatment for the couple equally. In another study, Guerra et al. (1998) found that psychiatric morbidity was considerably more pronounced in IVF-treated women and that this increased with the number of treatment cycles.

Patient satisfaction with care is now described as a priority area for care providers, and government policies are urging health trusts to examine their services (Christie, 1999). Hammarberg et al.'s (2001) follow-up study of women two to three years after ceasing treatment has shown that women who were unsuccessful were more critical of the clinic and the treatment received and were less satisfied with their life than those who were successful. However, other factors could have affected satisfaction. For example, in primary care, more time spent with GPs (Safran et al., 1998) and GPs' behaviour relate to greater satisfaction, as well as age, race and better-perceived health status, rather than differences in practice styles or specialities (Bertakis et al., 1998; Safran et al., 1998). Moreover, Holcomb et al. (1998) found that satisfaction was also related to perceived gains in diagnosis and treatment, which is likely to be relevant to assisted conception care. Smith et al. (2000) compared women who were currently still in treatment with women who were treated a year earlier. They found no differences in satisfaction with treatment between those questioned one year after treatment or those currently still in treatment, and no differences between those with a positive or negative outcome. One observation they made was that the outcome (failure, multiple births, and so on) had not met their expectations, suggesting that information regarding treatment outcome probabilities needs to be continually reinforced rather than given only at the start of treatment.

Considering the relatively low success rates of infertility treatments, the consequences of treatment failure need to be discussed prior to treatment and support, post-treatment, needs to be available. Freeman et al.'s (1987) study looked at the emotional responses of women who achieved pregnancy following treatment with those who failed, and compared these with women who withdrew of their own accord. Most of the women studied in this sample reported the treatment procedures as highly stressful (88% in the group who became pregnant and 83% in those who failed). However, **psychological dysfunction** was not evident in the long term, regardless of outcome. Furthermore, resolution was generally good in all groups, although those who did not take up the offer of subsequent treatment showed greater resolution to their childless status than both other groups.

Mao and Wood (1984) found that if individuals started treatment, and withdrew following one or more unsuccessful treatment cycles, the picture was rather more muddled. The financial burden was rated quite high as a reason for stopping treatment, as was the psycho-social stress of the procedures and repeated failure. However, resolution cannot have been very high in the group studied here, as the authors reported that 70% would consider re-entering the treatment programme again at some point in the future. The lack of resolution found in Mao and Wood's study has recently been confirmed by Strauss et al. (1998). They found that couples who terminated treatment after one year had higher interpersonal complaints and higher partner problems. This suggests that rather than terminating treatment because couples are able to resolve their infertility status, the conflicts experienced are worse rather than better. Bourguignon et al. (1998) studied 20 women two years after IVF failure and reported that 'the experience of IVF seems physically unintegrable. Propositions are made on contra-indications and pre-cautions to take before proposing IVF.' These studies suggest that counselling should precede and accompany the treatment throughout, and that it should also be provided post-treatment. Unfortunately, in practice we are a long way from providing this effectively in all cases.

Psychological side-effects from drugs taken during treatment have also been reported. Persaud and Lam (1998) observed a woman's psy-chologically extreme behaviour change following a manic reaction to gonadotropin administration to induce ovulation (see earlier in this chapter). Initially the woman displayed an elated mood and an increase in energy, sexual desire and activity. This was followed some two months later by clinical depression. She returned to make a good recovery following administration of a drug called Sertraline (used to treat depression). The authors speculate that this response may be more likely in people predisposed to depressive disorders, and suggest that this should be watched out for in women undergoing ovulation induction.

Another effect which has received research attention is the effect of infertility treatments on the children born from them. In 1990, Golombok et al. studied the emotions, social, psychosexual and cognitive development of children conceived by IVF. Overall, good progress was observed, although the incidence of behavioural and emotional problems in their sample exceeded that found in the non-IVF population.

Another issue, already given some attention, concerns that of donation of gametes for treatment. Although issues of donation are described in more detail elsewhere (Chaper 10), in oocyte donation, particularly if egg-sharing practices are used, it is important to note that a woman using her own oocytes for IVF who also shares the remainder with others undergoing IVF may fail her treatment. If the recipients succeed, this can have psychological consequences for the woman sharing her gametes, both at the time and a long way into the future. The HFEA Act (1990) gives any children born from donated gametes since 1990 the right to access non-identifying information about their genetic origin, once they have reached an appropriate age.

With further advances in treatment options there is an accompanying need for research. For example, interest has recently focused on a patient's interpretation of an embryo. The emotional effects of seeing an embryo transferred into the uterus can be great. A couple may be inclined to perceive this vision as their baby, even though rationally they know it is an embryo with a limited success rate for implantation. A report by a couple in a newsletter published by the self-help organisation CHILD (Anonymous, 1999) revealed the 'haunted' feelings a couple were left with after seeing their embryos on screen. In this case, the embryos failed to implant, and the effects of the knowledge that they had seen their prospective babies, and the familiarity and subsequent failure of implantation, was so devastating for this couple that they were moved to share their experiences in this newsletter. This indicates that any new intervention must be accompanied by a psychological assessment of the effects of the intervention, or of part of the technique, like a video representation. Professionals in infertility treatment should also be able to offer support in digesting the events appropriately. However, in many clinics such thorough care remains an undisputed necessity which may come into practice in the future.

FURTHER INFORMATION

Further information on treatments can be obtained from the sources listed below.

A total of 115 Clinics in the UK hold an HFEA licence for either assisted conception or donor insemination. It is not within the scope of this book to list them all, but details are available in a recent British Fertility Society article (see Balen, 1998).

The journal *Human Reproduction* has issued guidelines for good practice in IVF laboratories (Gianaroli et al., 2000). The embryology special interest group was responsible for drawing up these guidelines, to support and give guidance to laboratory staff. Interested readers should consult the journal.

Tavistock Marital Studies Institute
120 Belsize Lane
London NW3 5BA
Tel: 0207 435 7111
Fax: 0207 435 1080
Email: tmsi@tmsi.org.uk
www.tmsi.org.uk

World Wide Fertility Network
www.ferti.net

7 Surrogacy

Since the publication of the first few cases of **surrogacy** in the media in 1985, this once unusual practice has become familiar to most households in the UK. Needless to say, the way surrogacy is depicted in the media is immensely controversial. No one story is similar, and no one account gives the reader any idea of what is actually involved. The predominant picture is one of dislike for the practice.

However, surrogate motherhood is simply one way for a woman previously unable to bear children on her own to commission another woman to carry a baby for her. A **surrogate mother** is a woman who is prepared to become pregnant and carry a baby for someone else. The intention is to give the baby to the commissioning couple after delivery. The **commissioning mother** is a woman who, for one of many reasons, cannot conceive or carry a baby to term herself. It is important to understand that no woman would consider surrogacy an option if she herself were capable of carrying a baby. If she did, it would be considered a social surrogacy arrangement, which is not accepted in the UK and is not condoned by the British Medical Association (BMA, 1996). In the US, regulations take on a different shape from the UK. For example, recent newspaper articles have described a gay couple involved in a surrogacy case in a way which is not accepted in the UK (Hall, 2000; McLeod, 2000). First of all, the couple were two males; second, they were fertile. Both these factors are not considered sufficient to grant legal parenthood in the UK. The regulatory body of the HFEA rightly or wrongly states that both a mother and a father are necessary to provide a good environment for the child, and the fact that this couple were not infertile is further frowned upon in the UK. They demonstrate a case of social surrogacy, that is, surrogacy used to bring about a pregnancy and subsequently a child for social rather than medical reasons. Last but not least, it is against UK regulations to use fertility treatment centres to deliberately bring about the conception of a child of a particular sex. The gay couple in question both used their own sperm, and one man's sperm was filtered using computerised sensors to separate male sperm from female sperm (carrying the Y or X chromosome). The intention was to bring about one female embryo, while the other man's separated sperm produced a male.

Both embryos were implanted into a surrogate who delivered and relinquished a baby girl and boy to this couple.

Surrogacy can take on two quite different forms: one is called 'straight', 'partial' or **'genetic' surrogacy**; the other is called 'full', 'host', 'IVF' or **'gestational' surrogacy**. In genetic surrogacy, the surrogate mother is inseminated by the commissioning woman's husband's (or partner's) sperm, using DI as described in Chapter 6. She therefore fertilises her own egg and carries a baby which is genetically her own. In gestational surrogacy, the surrogate mother undergoes treatment at a clinic to have the commissioning couple's embryo transferred to her womb, using in vitro fertilisation (IVF) (also described in Chapter 6). Here the surrogate mother has no genetic link to the resulting baby, as she has not used her own egg. The complex possibilities in surrogacy are outlined in Table 7.1.

Table 7.1   Possible links with a baby in surrogacy

Link	Description
Commissioning mother	The woman who wants to have a child through surrogacy
Commissioning father	The man who wants to have a child through surrogacy
Surrogate mother or birth mother	The woman who agrees to conceive and carry a baby until delivery and relinquishes the baby to another woman following delivery
Genetic surrogate	The surrogate mother who conceives a baby using her own eggs and is inseminated (usually) with the commissioning father's sperm, who relinquishes the baby upon delivery
Gestational surrogate	The surrogate mother who agrees to undergo IVF treatment to carry the embryo of another couple to term, and relinquish the baby following delivery
Genetic mother	The woman who supplies the egg for the embryo. This could be a donor, the surrogate or the commissioning mother
Genetic father	The man who supplies the sperm for insemination or for the embryo. This could be a donor or the commissioning father
Social mother	The mother who raises and nurtures the child from birth as her own
Social father	The father who raises and nurtures the child from birth as his own

Approximately two-thirds of Britain's surrogate babies are conceived using genetic surrogacy, a less time- and money-consuming option with higher success rates than gestational surrogacy. However, the genetic option carries with it a greater risk of emotional distress for the surrogate who gives up her baby, for the commissioning mother who accepts a baby which is not genetically hers, and possibly for the child, who may have a closer early link with the surrogate, both gestationally and genetically, than with the commissioning mother fulfilling the social link. It is impossible to speculate on the relative importance of the gestational, genetic or social bonds between the mothers and children, but some reports tend to indicate that knowledge of the people involved, that is, 'openness', is less likely to have emotionally adverse consequences than anonymous arrangements between the parties involved or secrecy towards the child regarding his or her conceptional origins.

In the UK, the first time that the general public became aware of surrogacy was in the case of a young woman called Kim Cotton in 1985; prior to this no one had really heard of surrogate motherhood. Kim provoked outrage through publicly announcing her **surrogate pregnancy** and her intention to relinquish the baby (baby Cotton) upon delivery. The controversy was great, not only because this woman was prepared to give up a baby conceived through insemination, and was thus genetically linked to her, but also because she had received money to carry and give up the baby, which was her own (a sum of £6,500). Her fame was brought about through an American company who brokered the arrangement, although Kim carried and delivered the baby in the UK.

This was the beginning of surrogate motherhood as we know it today. Surrogacy has become increasingly recognised as an option for infertile couples, although it is still not accepted by many people. It has grown from nothing into a relatively widespread practice used by people from every corner of the country. A lot has happened since, progress has been made, the practice has become more formalised, and agencies have sprung up solely for the introduction of couples into surrogate arrangements. However, despite the tremendous efforts put into the operationalisation of UK surrogacy, the controversy surrounding it remains as intense as ever. There are fears today that surrogacy will disappear from the hands of the agencies and that it may, once again, become a frowned-upon practice, carried out by unscrupulous people for the sake of money. Box 7.1 outlines the processes involved in surrogacy as an option in overcoming childlessness.

Box 7.1   Processes involved in a surrogate arrangement

- Regardless of all other possible fertility problems in the man or woman, one prerequisite is that the woman has no possibility at all of carrying a baby to term. This can be because a congenital absence of the uterus, a previous hysterectomy or repeated miscarriages
- The couple can approach a surrogate agency directly or via a clinic
- The benefit of the route through a clinic is that medical monitoring and care will be provided in addition to that provided by the agency
- The disadvantage is that IUI carried out by a clinic is more expensive than if it is carried out 'at home'
- The agency will note the details and attempt to find a suitable surrogate
- The couple will be provided with information on procedures, costs and behaviour throughout the process, from meeting the surrogate to maintaining appropriate relationships during fertilisation, pregnancy and delivery
- The couple will be offered counselling
- The couple may then meet a surrogate and plan the arrangement
- In most cases telephone helpline support is available from the agency
- The surrogate baby will be registered on the birth certificate as the surrogate's baby, even if she made no genetic contribution to the child
- A Parental Order has to be sought to formally re-register the surrogate child as the child of the commissioning couple

---

In surrogacy, as indicated in Box 7.1, a certain amount of legal procedures are involved. If a surrogate carries a baby for another couple, the carrying mother is generally considered to be the legal mother, and her partner, the legal father of that child. The surrogate mother is obliged to register the birth of her child, and her partner (if she has one) normally becomes registered on the birth certificate as the father. The commissioning parents may become the **legal parents** of the child if they apply for **Parental Orders** (HFEA, Regulations 1994; HFEA, Scotland, Regulations). These allow parental rights and obligations to be transferred from the surrogate or birth parent(s) to the commissioning parents. The local Family Proceedings Courts (Magistrates Courts) hold the application forms, and in some cases Legal Aid may be available to cover the costs involved in the Parental Order proceedings. A number of conditions must be fulfilled prior to the application:

- The child must be genetically related to at least one of the two commissioning parents
- The surrogate parent(s) must consent to the making of the Order (which cannot be made before the child is six weeks old)
- The commissioning couple must be married and aged over 18
- The commissioning couple must apply for an order within the first six months of the child's birth
- Apart from expenses, there must be no other money exchanged between the commissioning and surrogate couples
- The child must be living with the commissioning couple
- The commissioning couple must live in the UK or the Channel Islands.

Once these conditions have been fulfilled, the application has been made and the Parental Order has been granted, the court Registrar-General will make the new entry in a separate Parental Order Register, re-registering the child. (Further information about Parental Orders can be obtained from the Department of Health.)

Even in cases where a close friend or family member is willing to be a surrogate, the commissioning parents need to ensure that they follow the same procedure as in cases where the surrogate and commissioning couple are complete strangers, in order to protect both parties involved. A surrogate will need counselling, because regardless of the quality of the relationship she may have with her commissioning relative or best friend, it may still be difficult to come to terms with relinquishing a baby. Legal processes must be carried out and, though not legally enforceable, a contract at the start of the arrangement can help both parties stick to the intended course of action. The following sections provide an outline of the wider psychological aspects of surrogacy, the organisations involved and the points of view of the commissioning mothers, the surrogates and the children.

PSYCHOLOGICAL AND SOCIAL ASPECTS OF SURROGACY

Little is known about the psychological or any other effects in relation to surrogacy. Although it has been a means of overcoming childlessness for the last decade or more in the UK, little research has been conducted to demonstrate the effects of this practice on those using it. What little research there is considers the effects on both the 'surrogate mother' and the 'commissioning mother'. (These will be discussed later on.) In the UK, one of the striking issues revealed about surrogacy concerns the importance some surrogates and commissioning women attach to a **genetic link** in a surrogate child. Snowden (1994) found that one genetic surrogate felt there was a child 'half mine walking around there somewhere'; another believed her gestational surrogacy was easier because the child was not genetically related to her and did not look like her or her own children. In my own studies on surrogacy, the same types of responses were received from both surrogate and commissioning women (van den Akker, 2000, 2001d). These issues need to be explored further in future research. Suffice it to say here, that whether a surrogate or a commissioning mother, genetic and gestational connections mean different things to different women.

The US has a much longer history of surrogacy and has produced a far greater amount of literature on surrogacy. However, because the processes involved in surrogacy are so different from those in the UK, it is not always possible to draw comparisons between British and American surrogate or commissioning couples.

SURROGATE MOTHERHOOD ORGANISATIONS

Surrogacy in the UK is very different from that in the US. In the US, companies employ surrogates and prescribe what they need to fulfil, how to do this and how much will be paid. A tough screening interview is generally carried out which includes a psychological assessment and medical examination. Much is asked about the potential surrogate's social life, her history and her anticipated future plans. If a surrogate does not meet all the criteria she may be rejected. In the UK, few of these processes are evident. Anyone can become a potential surrogate provided, in general, she has had at least one child of her own. Criteria, though discussed, are lenient, and no medical examination is needed. This in itself poses many threats to the commissioning couple, to the baby and to the surrogate herself. For example, the surrogate or the commissioning husband may be a carrier of a disease or genetic condition. Either way, upon reaching the age of 18 years the child can sue either party for damages if he or she is born with a disease or condition.

It is essential that both parties are aware of the risks they are taking, and crucial that these risks are minimised. It is partly for these reasons that the Minister for Health has commissioned a report into current practices, as **regulation** is desperately needed. Most clinics involved in IVF have stressed the need for a regulatory body to monitor the outcome for all involved in this practice. Agencies have also urged for regulation, and since they have the essential experience to demonstrate the particular areas within surrogacy that should be the focus for regulation it is surprising that so far little input from them has been accepted.

Two of my recent studies have attempted to document the functions of professional involvement and have evaluated the type of assessments clinics and organisations dealing with surrogacy use to determine the suitability of surrogate and commissioning mothers. In 1998 a number of clinics and agencies in Britain involved with surrogacy were interviewed about their practices. Only ten centres were interviewed, because although many more clinics had a great interest in surrogacy, they had not yet obtained an HFEA licence or had not started a surrogate IVF pregnancy. Only agencies and clinics 'experienced' with surrogacy were therefore interviewed.

The data presented in Table 7.2 show the enormous demand for surrogacy and the type of responsibility taken on by the clinics and agencies. It is clear that, considering the number of enquiries, the demand for the service appears to be out of proportion to the small number of organisations trying to meet that demand. Interestingly, recruitment of surrogates is not done by clinics but indirectly by agencies. There are clear reasons for this. Clinics are not allowed to find a surrogate for a commissioning client, and agencies are not allowed to advertise for them. Compared to American practices, therefore, it is surprising that any form of system manages to survive in the UK.

In practice very few surrogate or commissioning women were rejected at any one time. The interviews carried out with the organisations involved in surrogacy in Britain have shown that each has put an enormous amount of effort into providing a means to assist infertile people through surrogacy within the constraints of the present legislation. The future of surrogacy, from an organisational perspective, could be improved if legislation were to change. This

Table 7.2 Characteristics of organisations involved in surrogacy between 1988 and 1998

	Agencies	Clinics
Years in practice with surrogacy	4–10 years	5–10 years
Means of approach for surrogates	Through the media	Through agencies
Numbers of commissioning mothers making enquiries	300–8,000	18–60
Numbers of surrogates making enquiries	200–600	0
Responsibility of determining suitability of surrogate and commissioning mother	In-house 'ethics' committee	Ethics committees, but often self-selected and self-constituted
Assistance provided to 'get to know' one another	Guidelines provided	Not specified in 4 out of 6 clinics
Counselling provision	Offered to all, but provision is ad hoc. Guidelines stipulate the number of sessions recommended	Offered, but provision is ad hoc
Specific information provided	Detailed written information/guidelines	Written clinic information provided. If counsellors are part of the team, specific surrogacy information is also given
Medical or psychological problems with commissioning mothers	0	1
Legal problems with commissioning mothers	0	0
Medical or psychological problems with surrogates	0	4
Legal problems with surrogates	2	1
Need for regulation	Yes	Yes

may not be possible until population attitudes reflect a better understanding of the practice.

Selection and assessment of surrogate and commissioning couples tends to be stringent and thorough in the US. In Britain, this is minimal. There are concerns that no one takes responsibility for assessing the parties involved in surrogacy. In 1999 I described the results of the same organisations interviewed for the 1998 study. In that paper I explored questions of responsibility in surrogacy. The majority of approaches for surrogacy come from heterosexual couples. Two clinics and one agency would not support gay or lesbian surrogacies because they considered it 'unethical' or illegal. Those reporting illegality as a reason for rejection are right, because it would constitute a social surrogacy, which is not accepted in the UK. However, those considering homosexual surrogacy to be unethical are exercising personal opinion, and this should be not be condoned. In terms of further assessment of their clients, 75% rated the surrogate and commissioning couple's knowledge about the practice as poor. This is not surprising, because little access to information is available until approaches are made. Few criteria for selection or assessment were stipulated. Only three clinics employed their own counsellors, while neither of the agencies did. Although this is partly a consequence of finances, it has an inadvertent effect on the quality of counselling the clients will receive. If expert counselling cannot be guaranteed then selection and assessment will invariably suffer. This could then lead to the involvement of inappropriate surrogates or commissioning mothers.

Some form of screening was carried out by all organisations, although their methods differed greatly. Furthermore, if an individual is rejected by one organisation, there is no mechanism in place preventing that person from trying another organisation; this has been known to happen. All organisations used some form of ethical committee to help in their selection procedures, and specific legal and psychological help was sought if it was deemed necessary. In short, only one clinic used in-depth psychological assessments, and assessments across organisations were not uniform. Bias in selection or rejection is likely to be taking place, although few people are rejected outright.

In summary, agencies and clinics involved with surrogacy operate within restrictions imposed by current regulations, some of which are not entirely reasonable and not evidence-based. On the other hand, erring on the side of caution is probably the best course of action. The practice could be improved if assessment, selection and payment were standardised, protected and legitimised in the future. Nevertheless, surrogacy in Britain works.

SURROGATE MOTHERS

Since surrogacy is such an unorthodox event, natural questions to ask would include: 'What sort of people are surrogates'?, 'What does it take to be a surrogate'?, and 'What are their motivations'? The only way to answer these questions is to ask women who have been surrogates. Much has been published in the media about the appalling characteristics of surrogate mothers, and in some cases they have been correctly described. However, these are the women who make it to press, and their reasons for talking to the media may be motivated by aspects unrelated to their actual surrogacy experiences. There are many more surrogates who have not been involved with the media, and it is perhaps these women who should provide the answers to the questions posed. Cotton (1985) has written an in-depth account of her experiences as a genetic and gestational surrogate which, unlike the media accounts, gives a good insight into surrogacy from the point of view of Britain's first surrogate mother.

Recent research and interviews with surrogates has helped in the development of some understanding of the characteristics and motivations of surrogate mothers (van den Akker, 2001d). Although the studies are in their early stages, some information is consistently revealed. What is perhaps the most easily answered question, and one that is answered adamantly and knowledgeably by most surrogates, is that they firmly believe that surrogacy takes a special type of person, and that not everyone is suitable to be a surrogate. Similarly, most surrogates seem to know if they can or cannot be a genetic surrogate, that is, if they can or cannot relinquish a baby which is genetically theirs. Some surrogates may be misleading themselves and choose on the basis of the medical interventions involved, or anticipated differences in money paid to them. Others may be too young to understand the consequences of their actions, or may think they do and then regret their decision later upon the time of relinquishment, or even later in life when it is too late to do anything about it.

American research has helped to provide some insight into what sort of people surrogates are. In particular, Helena Ragone (1994) has written a detailed account of her interviews and discussions with surrogate mothers. Ragone insists that one cannot even begin to look at surrogacy without examining the 'role of women's work and the separation of domestic work from the public sphere' (p51). She argues that the relevance of the separation of the home and the workplace after the industrial revolution marked the separation of the domestic and public spheres. Surrogacy, she argues, bridges that gap between the public and domestic arenas (p52). Her conclusions refer to surrogates as women willing to 'give the gift of life'. Other writers have exemplified the woes of surrogacy through dwelling on the **commodification** of women's procreative abilities. Those attributes, particularly in paid or **commercial surrogacy**, have been described as being a threat to socio-economically deprived women. Less well off or less well educated women may use their bodies for financial reward. Through paid reproduction they may be challenging the constitution of motherhood, the mother–child bond, and the nuclear family structure.

Blyth (1994), and more recently, I (van den Akker, 2001d) have described British surrogate mothers' feelings and experiences of surrogacy. Blyth interviewed 19 surrogates, while I asked 15 surrogates to complete long questionnaires. The women studied were very similar in socio-economic, educational, age and parity terms. None of them were particularly well off. A few surrogates explicitly stated that money was one reason for becoming a surrogate, although the majority said they did this for **altruistic** reasons. Most surrogates enjoyed pregnancy and childbirth, and interestingly many surrogates said that surrogacy fulfilled or added something to their lives. These responses refer to increased feelings of self-worth, self-confidence, the development of intense and unusual friendships with the commissioning parents (particularly the commissioning mothers) and the feeling that they had done something worthwhile with their lives. (The title of Eric Blyth's 1994 paper reflects this: 'I wanted to be interesting. I wanted to be able to say "I've done something interesting with my life."'.) **Relinquishment** of the baby was a happy event for most surrogates. Many explained that their happiness came from seeing the face of the commissioning mother when they first held the baby, others said they felt relief that it was all over. Happiness was mixed with sadness during relinquishment for a proportion of the women.

The surrogates from both studies unequivocally said that they believed the commissioning mothers should disclose the arrangement to their surrogate child(ren). None of the surrogates felt exploited, and all said they expected the commissioning parents to be truthful and open about the child's origins, as they told all their own children about the surrogate baby. The majority expected some contact between them to continue following relinquishment of the baby, and in some cases this ceased unexpectedly after the legal proceedings had been completed. The long-term care and support of the surrogate mother is not necessarily first and foremost in the commissioning couple's mind. Some surrogates have reported that they were surprised by these 'selfish' attitudes; others reported this as showing a lack of concern for the surrogate's own children. Many surrogates involve their own family in the surrogacy process. This makes it easier for their children to understand what is involved and to know about the couple who will have their mother's 'tummy baby'. It is seen as betrayal when the commissioning couple with the surrogate baby suddenly disappear from the surrogate's and her family's life.

Although most surrogates said they would do it again, there were some who said that they definitely would not. In Blyth's study, one surrogate could not give the commissioning couple the baby. This was not because she wanted the baby, but because she developed concerns about the commissioning couple and felt that 'she was not prepared to entrust the care of the baby to them'. Lastly, although genetic and gestational surrogate arrangements are utterly different, in terms of psychological functioning I found few differences between them on standardised assessment scales (van den Akker, 2001d). In the longer term, however, differences may well emerge, because, as Blyth pointed out, gestational surrogates benefit from the 'full panoply of regulation (as it is)' involving organisational control and support provisions, while genetic surrogates operate 'in a moral and psychological twilight' in which participants are left very much to their own devices. The future of surrogacy in Britain will benefit from more adequate screening of both surrogate and commissioning couples, to avoid disappointment on either part. Research should be carried out to determine the immediate and long-term effects of surrogacy on the surrogate mother, and on her own children. It is only with evidence-based guidelines that practice can be supported and improved.

COMMISSIONING MOTHERS

For infertile couples seeking a surrogate's help to have a baby, things tend to be, initially at least, not as 'exciting' an option as it can be interpreted for surrogates. Women opting for surrogacy tend to be women who do not have a uterus or womb (usually the result of a hysterectomy), have **congenital** abnormalities of the womb, or in a few cases they may be women who cannot maintain a pregnancy. In the UK, surrogacy is only accepted as an alternative means of having a baby if medical reasons indicate that this is the only option. In other words, it tends to be chosen as a last resort.

Surrogacy is an alternative to adoption, but differs in that it allows for some genetic link with the child. If the male is in a position to use his own gametes, these will either be used through artificial insemination with the surrogate mother, or they will be fertilised in vitro with his partner's (the commissioning woman's) egg. Thus either a full or partial genetic link is possible in surrogacy. There are a few cases where no genetic link to either the commissioning mother or father is used, but such cases are rare in the UK. Other aspects which can be seen as advantages of surrogacy over adoption include the fact that the commissioning couple take home a newborn baby, as opposed to a child, and the commissioning mother could, if she so desired, attempt to breastfeed the baby (Biervliet et al., 2001).

The commissioning of a surrogate baby has been seen as a challenge to what constitutes a family and reproduction. It secures the fragmentation of reproductive functioning in several ways:

- it separates sex from reproduction
- it separates motherhood from pregnancy
- it separates the unity of one couple into the involvement of a third person within the potential family relationship.

These factors, unique to commissioning a surrogate baby, do not need to result in a confusion of family or of belonging. Psychologists have investigated the effect the lack of or ambiguous genetic and biological relationships between parents and children in families created through surrogacy may have, and what characterises people who opt for surrogacy. In a study of 29 women commissioning a surrogate baby, I found that the main reason for considering having a surrogate baby was that 'it was the only way for us to have a child' (just over half the women did not have a uterus). Other reasons were because they would have a full or partial genetic link with the child (something not possible with adoption), or because IVF or adoption failed (van den Akker, 2000).

As with any option to overcome childlessness, this one is not without risks or worries. One of the risks involved is the possibility of ovarian hyperstimulation syndrome (see Chapter 6) in commissioning women hoping to use their own egg for in vitro fertilisation and transfer of the embryo to the surrogate mother. Another risk involves any condition a genetic surrogate (who uses her own egg) might pass on to the commissioned child. Fears include the fact that the surrogate may not relinquish the baby, and even some fears of **social stigma** towards a commissioning couple or their surrogate child (van den Akker, 2000). It is also possible that there may be problems identified in the offspring once they realise that their mother either did not carry them or is in fact genetically not their mother. However, although no studies have been carried out on the children commissioned through surrogacy (many of them are still very young), no adverse affects appear to have shown themselves, according to the commissioning mothers themselves. Furthermore, all commissioning women studied in the UK by Blyth (1995) and myself (2000) have said that they would never hide the fact that the child was carried by a surrogate, from their child or anyone else.

Few psychological studies have been carried out in the UK on commissioning mothers, and even less is available on the fathers. In general, both Blyth's (1995) and my results (2000) noted that surrogacy was largely initiated through information from the media, based on gut feelings in the matching process between the commissioning mother and her surrogate, and based on trust between the couples or individuals concerned. Trust was a two-way phenomenon, with the surrogate trusting the commissioning couple to pay the fee, and the commissioning couple trusting the surrogate to care for the baby in utero and relinquish it upon delivery.

In 1995, Blyth reported that a minority of his study group were using IVF or gestational surrogacy, with the majority opting for genetic or DI surrogacy. In 2000, however, the picture was reversed with a small majority of my sample opting for gestational surrogacy (n = 16) and a minority opting for genetic surrogacy (n = 13). Although this shift in type of surrogacy used suggests a change in availability of IVF surrogacy, it must be borne in mind that in my study, all women explained that they opted for the gestational route because they could use their own egg. The reverse was true for most of the women opting for genetic surrogacy (although a few chose this for financial reasons, surrogate preference or because the gestational option had already failed). It is also likely that as both

Blyth's and my samples were based on individuals volunteering to take part in these studies, self-selection could account for these differences, because in statistical terms the majority of surrogate arrangements are reported to be genetic surrogacy arrangements (van den Akker, 1998a).

Interestingly, both of these studies observed that the importance of a genetic link was largely based on pragmatism. If they were in a position to use their own genetic material the majority reported it was important. Conversely, if gestational surrogacy was not an option, they tended to report that a genetic link was not important. Both studies also report an overwhelming intent on the part of the commissioning mothers to inform their child(ren) that they were brought into the world through surrogacy; a finding that contrasts the views held by recipients of donor gametes.

Another important observation made in both these studies was that commissioning mothers were not inclined to attempt to justify their unusual choice. Virtually all the women studied were able to reconcile the difference of a surrogate family with other families. They did not feel the need to deny their choice, and did not feel the need to deny their differences. These results were interesting because there was a decline in public support for surrogacy (Brook et al., 1992; Halman et al., 1992), and little acceptance of the practice in general (ICM Research, 1994). The majority of commissioning mothers in my study revealed that they intended to maintain some contact with their surrogate (van den Akker, 2000). They referred to this contact as 'Christmas card contact', that is, once a year they would be exchanging a card saying they were well. These expectations were quite different for a proportion of the surrogates discussed earlier.

SURROGATE BABIES

Although some research has been carried out on the adults involved in surrogate motherhood, little is known about the children brought about as a result of surrogacy. There are now at least several hundred children born as a result of surrogate arrangements in the UK (van den Akker, 1998a). This figure is likely to be larger, because not all surrogate and commissioning couples feed back to the agencies if and when they successfully complete these arrangements. It is also likely that arrangements have taken place outside of any involvement of organisations involved in surrogacy, making accurate documentation impossible. The surrogate children born in the UK are all roughly under the age of 16. The majority are still very young and therefore unable to voice their opinions on what it is like for them to be a surrogate child, or how they feel about their genetic or gestational 'mother'. These views will no doubt become public in the next few years, and they should help to provide a framework for future practice.

Unlike many other ways of creating families, the parents of surrogate children tend to be open about their conception, gestation and genetic origins. This is in part because many surrogate and commissioning couples develop a strong bond or friendship during the arrangements as both physical and emotional changes are relevant to both parties. Many couples also experience tremendous ups and downs, for example, the joy when the result of a pregnancy test is positive and the experience of birth is shared, or if a pregnancy has not been established or results in a miscarriage then both parties suffer together under these intimate conditions. They therefore get to know each other well and most intend to keep in contact well after the arrangement has terminated. The child then refers to the surrogate as an aunt or 'other' mum (or even a 'tummy mum').

Telling a child the truth about his or her origins can be very difficult for the parents. This can be more difficult if it is left until later on in the child's life. Yet we know from people who were adopted or conceived using donor sperm or eggs that most would like to know about their origins, and if possible they would like to get to know their 'genetic' parent(s) (Dudley and Neave, 1997; Howe and Feast, 2000). In surrogacy the same applies. Surrogate conceptions are unusual, but not uncommon. There are fears of social stigma on the part of some parents (van den Akker, 2000), and fears about who the true genetic parent(s) of the child are. For example, I found that some commissioning mothers reported that they were concerned about the test tubes being mixed up, or the surrogate husband's sperm having fertilised the surrogate rather than the commissioning husband's inseminated sperm. These are all reasonable fears and can be allayed using genetic testing. However, assuming all fertilisation was carried out with the chosen genes, it could be difficult to tell a child over a certain age that his or her mum did not really carry him or her, or that in fact he or she is the child of another mother and the current dad. This could have devastating consequences for a child, and should be avoided. Until surrogate children are old enough to understand the issue, simply keeping the debate open is the only option, although we should be wise enough to draw on the experiences of the now grown adult people conceived through other means. Their views or needs may not be identical, but they are more likely to be comparable.

Having seen many surrogate children at annual meetings of COTS (Childlessness Overcome Through Surrogacy), there was no indication at all that any of them had suffered as a result of the knowledge they had acquired at an early age about their unusual origins. Accounts of commissioning mothers show that most intend to tell their children from an early age how they were conceived and carried. Linda Nelson, a commissioning mother of twins, tells her story of openness and honesty not only toward her children, but the wider social network. She says 'I have not been aware of any change in other people's attitude towards the twins, which would be my only concern' (Nelson, 1998). From the point of view of the children's knowledge of their origins, Nelson notes: 'I can only hope that, as they grow up, they will understand our struggle to bring them into the world.' Nelson is unusual, because not only could she not carry a pregnancy to term and used a surrogate to carry her and her husband's embryo's, she also donated eggs herself to another infertile couple. In this latter case, she again advocated honesty about this child's genetic origins. The daughter born from Linda's egg now lives abroad, but she has had progress reports and early photographs of the child, and the parenting couple have agreed to be truthful to the child about her genetic mother. In fact, although disclosure is clearly the preferred option in the considerably older practice of adoption, in surrogacy, most clinics insist that egg donation should be done anonymously. This is not based on evidence of donated offspring's wishes (Howe and Feast, 2000) but to ensure that prospective donors continue to come forward. However, little effort has been expended in the UK in addressing these issues adequately with the relevant regulatory bodies such as the HFEA, BMA or hospital ethics committees.

Another account of the benefits of openness of origins comes from surrogates. The most recent examples of surrogates' experiences of relinquishing a genetic or gestational baby under relatively open or 'closed' conditions comes from Cheryl Davis and Kim Cotton. Both were surrogates and both relinquished their babies to other couples. Kim Cotton's recent revelations about her first genetic surrogate baby produced some heart-rending truths about the disadvantages of 'closed' or anonymous surrogacy. Kim did not get to know the couple, and had no contact with the baby following relinquishment. She herself now admits that this can have 'barbaric' consequences for the surrogate, and can be as dramatically perceived by the child once he or she finds out. She wrote a book about both her surrogacy experiences, and felt at the time that she was young, inexperienced and 'dictated' to with the first one. Kim Cotton has recently resigned from her role as Chair of COTS, Britain's main surrogate agency, and gave an emotional interview in the *Mail on Sunday*. Here she told how the first experience now appears devastating, and how she is troubled by the thought of the child she never knew. The same concerns were voiced by Cheryl Davies.

Kim's second surrogacy experience was completely different. In the second case, she knew the commissioning mother well before offering herself as her surrogate. They still see each other and each other's families, and the emotional turmoil in this case is absent. It is likely that the lack of a genetic link between the second surrogacy arrangement (producing twins) and the first also made a difference to her ability to cope with the relinquishment. In fact Linda Nelson (personal communication, 1998) wrote an account of how one of her surrogate twins relates to Kim, their surrogate mother: 'It was a good job we had Kim as your friend, mummy. Otherwise you wouldn't have us.' This comment came from a seven-year-old surrogate child, and shows no signs of ill-effects whatsoever. Linda brought her up knowing her gestational origins and Kim, the surrogate, openly. Both parties are satisfied with the children's behaviour, reactions and understanding, and neither the surrogate nor the commissioning mother has any regrets about the arrangement, but share the joy of the children they jointly brought into this world.

FURTHER INFORMATION

A number of texts specifically on surrogacy abroad are listed below, which will provide some insight into the sort of people who become surrogates or use surrogacy. However, it must be borne in mind that their experiences will be different as a result of the American legislative and medical systems.

For further information on American systems see the following publications.

Helena Ragone (1994)
Surrogate Motherhood: Conception in the Heart
Westview Press, Boulder, CO

Gail Dutton (1997)
A Matter of Trust: The Essential Guide to Gestational Surrogacy
Clouds Publishing, California

Cheryl Saban (1998)
Miracle Child: Genetic Mother, Surrogate Womb
New Horizon Press, Far Hills, NJ

Elaine Gordon (1992)
Mommy, Did I Grow in Your Tummy? Where Some Babies Come From
Em Greenberg, Santa Monica, CA

Herbert Richardson (ed.) (1987)
On the Problem of Surrogate Motherhood: Analysing the Baby M Case
Edwin Mellen, New York/Ontario

Cheryl Shalev (1989)
The Case for Surrogacy
Yale University Press, New Haven, CT

Further information about aspects of surrogacy can be obtained from the organisations listed below.

Surrogacy Agencies

COTS
(Childlessness Overcome Through Surrogacy)
Secretary: Gena Dodd
Loandhu Cottage
Gruids
Lairg
Sutherland
IV27 4EF
COTS information line: 0906 680 0088
Email: cotsuk@enterprise.net

www.surrogacy.org.uk

SPC
(Surrogate Parenting Centre)
2 Woodland Court
Shenstone Woodend
Staffordshire WS14 0PE
Tel: 0121 323 3156

www.surrogacy.com

Parental Orders

Department of Health
Health Promotion Division
Room 417
Wellington House
133–155 Waterloo Road
London SE1 8UG
Tel: 0207 972 2000

8   Adoption

Adoption is definitely a possibility for some infertile couples who will not be able to achieve parenthood in any other way. This could be one way of becoming a parent on a permanent basis. There are many couples who have been accepted and are waiting for adoption. In the past, applicants who were still undergoing fertility treatment were not assessed for adoption until they had completed their treatment. This is now changing. Unlike the procedures discussed in Chapter 6, where the aim is to find or obtain a pregnancy or baby for the infertile couple, in adoption the opposite occurs: the children are there and the aim of adoption agencies is to find parents for these children.

There are different ways of going about adopting a child, and different requirements are needed for some of these. Adoption is subject to the 1989 Children Act and the 1976 Adoption Act. All adoption agencies abide by regulations laid out in these acts. The British Association for Adoption and Fostering (BAAF) has compiled a large database of many adoption issues. For example, it has a database of members, which are all voluntary and local authority agencies dealing with adoption; and a database of research into adoption. BAAF also provides its own information about adoption in its publications.

Information changes rapidly, and it is therefore necessary at all times to ensure that information is always up to date. (Comprehensive material providing more detailed information concerning the changes in adoption issues, trends and controversies, can be found in Hill and Shaw, 1998.) Furthermore, all agencies' statutory work is dependent on local conditions. For example, an agency in one particular area may need to focus on finding parents for black or Muslim children; while others may focus entirely on older children.

Adoption of children already existing is declining. For many children seeking adoptive parents, more parents than children exist. This is not the case for children with severe problems, both mental and physical, and for those with serious handicaps or children from abroad. Children available for adoption also tend to be older, with few healthy infants or young children available for adoption placement. The reasons for this are in part because of better **contraceptive** availability, an increase in abortions and a decrease in negative social stigma for young or unmarried mothers.

Consequently, the adoption option may be time-consuming and may not always result in the type of parenting infertile couples initially envisaged. Nevertheless, adoption practices have advanced in recent years. Adoptive children are placed in families faster than used to be the case, and their time in care tends to be shorter. Adoption agencies now also emphasise the placing of adoptive children in families matching their own socio-cultural and **ethnic backgrounds**. Another change in practice today is that adoption has moved from a 'closed' to an 'open' process. Where **anonymity** was maintained in the past, all parties are now aware of each other. This is to ensure that the adoptive children feel secure within their new families, but also that they can maintain contact with important people from their past. Adoption agencies recognise the need to accept the importance of the ability to care over the need to be in traditional family set-ups. For example, single, gay, lesbian and older people are given the opportunity to adopt. What is essential in adoption is that the prospective parents are able to provide a stable, caring home for children. This is a requirement of 'parental responsibility', no matter how the child ended up in a particular family. Ultimately, the need for a child is so great in so many people, that the opportunity to adopt a child will be taken, no matter the difficulties.

Clearly, to be considered for adoption, a person does not need to be infertile, unlike in surrogacy, where this practice is legally allowed only if no alternatives are possible. Single, gay or lesbian people are not socially in a position to have children, and hence have to be excluded from surrogacy arrangements. In adoption and fostering these limitations are much more relaxed to accommodate the needs of many, particularly older, children.

When an individual enquires about the possibility of adopting a child, the agency's main concern is for the welfare of the child to be placed. In fact legislation and adoption agencies' procedures are informed largely by the children's needs. In other words, the family has to be right for the child, not vice versa. Many adoptions are the result of social care interventions. The implications of this are that many parents do not necessarily consent to having their child(ren) adopted. Adoption agencies now make it clear to prospective parents that many of their children have been subject to deprived environments, neglect or even abuse. Abused children include those subjected to multiple foster homes and who are, as a result of those moves, 'unintentionally' abused. The prospect of taking on a child who may have suffered any form of physical or emotional trauma is daunting to many prospective parents. It is exactly for these reasons that some form of suitability assessment of adoptive parents is also essential to ensure that a good environment can be provided and that the needs of these children can be met.

Overseas adoption is not necessarily an easier option for prospective parents. Many children or infants placed for adoption overseas will have suffered deprivation of one sort or another. Moreover, it is less likely that accurate information about their background and medical histories will be available. This can have implications for the appropriate placement of these children, because adequate matching may not be possible. A recent dispute in the media has highlighted a difficult and unusual case involving overseas adoption (Branigan and Carter, 2001), though the difficulties were unrelated to the matching process. A British couple 'bought' American baby twins via the internet. That in itself was newsworthy, but the case was complicated by the twins having already been 'sold' to another couple in the US. The couple paying the most money – the British couple – eventually took the babies home. Since baby-buying is not condoned the case was referred to the Home Office, and unfortunately for all parties concerned, the twins are still in temporary care at the time of writing. The processes involved in adoption are outlined in Box 8.1.

As described in Box 8.1, an individual or couple who feel they want to pursue this option need to be realistic about the adoption agencies assessment procedures, which can be lengthy (Chennells and Hammond, 1998). Initially there are some checks which need to be made. This can put many people off, but considering the welfare of the child is at stake, this is probably not unreasonable. Police and local authority checks, and medical and personal references are undertaken. These can take several months because a number of different organisations are involved. Criteria for unsuitability based on the above checks are generally stringent. For example, if it comes to light that one member of a family applying for adoption has a Schedule 1 conviction (an offence involving violence against a child), the family is immediately ruled out for adoption. Agencies may use their own discretion if other offences come to light. Relationship factors such as previous relationship break-ups, previous abortions, and medical factors such as unstable mental health or a life-threatening illness, can also constitute reasons for rejection.

> **Box 8.1   Processes involved in adoption**
>
> - Initial enquiries can be directed at social services or listed adoption agencies around the country
> - The couple will be asked to complete preliminary forms
> - The couple will be interviewed regarding motivations for adopting and suitability for adoption
> - A number of checks will be made, such as police and local authority checks
> - Medical references will be sought
> - Personal references will be sought
> - In-depth interviews will be undertaken
> - Regular visits will be made
> - Meetings with other prospective adoptive applicants and with people successful at adoption will be set up
> - Suitability assessments will be carried out
> - If successful, a formal letter of acceptance will be issued
> - The services or agency will then start a matching process between a possible child and the couple

Following these initial checks, **in-depth interviews** are conducted with the prospective adoptive parent(s), which can take well over three months. These take the form of regular visits from adoption agency representatives to the prospective adopters' house, and visits by the prospective adopters to the agencies. Many interviews will be conducted between the representative and the prospective parents, with both partners of a couple together and on their own. In addition meetings are set up to prepare the applicants for the reality of adoption. This includes meeting other people at the same stage in the adoption application process, meeting former adoptive parents and adult adoptees, and preparing for the numerous issues which need to be addressed within a prospective adoptive family such as health and disclosure needs, and questions about genetic and cultural heritage. Most of the individuals concerned enjoy this aspect of the process thoroughly, particularly meeting other prospective adoptive parents (van den Akker, 2001a). Within these meetings, the focus moves away from the individual and adoption is seen in a wider, shared context.

Following this long process to ensure that adoptive parents have been thoroughly checked and are properly prepared for the difficulties they may face with adoptive children, the process of acceptance or rejection takes place. Usually a specially set up panel reports on the applicants' suitability. They will decide if that particular placement for adoption is in the child's best interest. Other important issues addressed at this stage concern the removal of parental rights. This is a matter for the courts and can be contested by the parents. If the panel accepts the applicants, and the child's parents' rights are completely removed, a formal letter of acceptance will be issued to the applicants. This letter will outline the number and type of children they have been approved for. There is then a period of matching a suitable child or children with the accepted adoptive parents, involving the prospective adoptive parents and the panel. BAAF publishes an inside guide to good practice of panels (Lord et al., 1997). Although this is a book written for panel members, it may be useful to find out what the new adoption panel regulations and policies are, so that individuals entering the adoption process can be well prepared.

It is important to note that once the panel is involved, it is unlikely that the applicants are rejected for adoption. However, once accepted, they may still have to wait for a considerable length of time for a suitable child to be found. Some agencies do not have children waiting to be placed for adoption, and this can result in stress for the accepted parents. BAAF provides an inter-agency service link which allows the opportunity to match parents with children throughout the country. However, the adoption process from start to finish can take as little as one year or as long as twelve years (van den Akker, 2001a).

PSYCHOLOGICAL AND SOCIAL ASPECTS OF ADOPTION

Much has been written about the psychological and social aspects of adoption. The **birth mothers**, the adoptive parent(s) and the children will be affected by adoption, and serious consideration has therefore been given to each of these. In 1996, David Howe wrote extensively about the experiences of adoptive parents, describing how people feel towards birth mothers, biology, infertility and parenting. Others (for example, Howe et al., 1997) focus on the feelings and emotions experienced by the birth mothers relinquishing their child for adoption. They describe the explicit social stigma associated with giving up a child; an area worth exploring for anyone considering this avenue as a means of overcoming childlessness. Perhaps the most important factor to consider when opting for adoption is the child. Again, numerous books have been written about helping children with the changes taking place around them, and their emotional, social and cultural needs.

Jewett's (1995) sensitively written book, *Helping Children Cope with Separation and Loss*, explores the grieving experienced through **case histories** of children who leave their birth home (accounts provided by individuals, and transcribed by the author). It is an area that needs special consideration, because nothing is more important than the well-being of any child. In fact, a recent increase in interest has focused on **post-adoption** issues for the child and the adopting and relinquishing parents. Most people involved in the adoption process need some form of support; some would argue that anyone setting up home with any new child or baby could do with support! This need is now well recognised, and although practical support is still scanty, the aim is to improve the services available, to increase understanding and to ensure benefits for all those in the post-adoption stage.

For the adoptive parents, a number of important 'steps' need to be taken before and during the adoption process. First, it is important to recognise that a biological child will not be forthcoming, and this has been termed the 'decision-making phase' (Hajal and Rosenberg, 1991). During this stage, the couple need to come to terms with this fact, and only when that is done can they safely consider the option of adoption. If this has not been consolidated, there is a danger that the yearning for a biological child could get in the way of accepting the adopted child as their own. This could lead to a fear that the adopted child is seen as a second-best alternative to the real thing, a genetic baby. The issue of being approved by an adoption agency is likely to have an effect on the couple, both psychologically and within their social environment. Unlike the case of birthing parents, in adoption, screening of motivations and competence can affect psychological functioning. For example, the process can be seen as invasive and feelings of guilt and inadequacy, particularly if the prospective adopters are rejected, are common.

Hobday and Lee (1995) discuss the research on a 'psychological pregnancy' after a child is offered to a prospective adoptive couple. This would give the prospective parents time to prepare and plan for the arrival of a child, and to prepare family and friends for this new addition to their family. Currently, little preparatory time and information is available for future adoptive parents (Dubois, 1987) despite the length of time spent waiting for a child. Once a child is adopted, there is a need for the parents and child to bond. Early psychological work on parents and their infants has stressed the importance of bonding in early life, for good psychological adjustment in later life (Bowlby, 1969; Rutter, 1981). Hajal and Rosenberg (1991) have described a phenomenon called the shadow of the birth parent hovering over the adoptive family, affecting the formation of bonds. In order to overcome the interference of such birth-parent shadows in the minds of the adoptive family, some form of help could be offered. When children are placed for adoption after their first few years, there may be some conflict in providing a secure, warm, dependable environment, and in the child's age-related need for independence and the need to develop a sense of his or her own identity. These issues are likely to be more pronounced in the adoption of older children, particularly adolescents. Most families bringing up biologically related adolescents have difficulty coming to terms with the dramatic changes taking place in the adolescent's external appearance and behaviour. Adoptive parents should accept this as a relative norm and not as something necessarily specific to the fact that their child is adopted. Again the need for professional help and understanding should not be underestimated, and this is currently recognised by psychological clinicians and researchers (Brodzinsky, 1987). I designed a study to determine if different processes to overcome childlessness had an effect on the psychological functioning of women opting for adoption, surrogacy or IVF treatment (van den Akker, 2001c). The results revealed that adopting mothers are not marked by increased anxiety or depression and do not have significantly more psychopathology than women opting for IVF or surrogacy. Quality of life was also comparable in the women studied who opted for disparate means to overcome their childlessness.

Research regarding the different choices available to people in their attempts to have a child varies. In 1997, van Balen et al. interviewed 131 infertile couples in the Netherlands (van Balen et al., 1997c). They found that the vast majority immediately decided to try a medical treatment option in an attempt to overcome childlessness. In contrast, alternative options such as adoption and fostering were considered only later. By then, the reasons for choosing adoption, and particularly fostering, were predominantly altruistic. I found that the medical option was considered seriously by the majority of the 105 participants studied. However, once they had decided on adoption, 41% chose this for altruistic reasons, 36% simply because it would provide them with a family, 11% because it would be a permanent solution, and 3% because it was the only remaining option for them. There was a proportion who believed that a genetic link (not obtained in adoption) held some importance for them. It is these cases who may not feel sufficiently resolved about the lack of their own genetic child, and who should probably consider adoption after a longer period of thought. No one child should be brought into a family if there is even the smallest possibility of that child being seen as a second-best option.

FURTHER INFORMATION

Further information about adoption can be obtained from the following organisations.

BAAF
(British Association for Adoption and Fostering)
Head Office
Skyline House
200 Union Street
London SE1 0LY
Tel: 0207 593 2000
Fax: 0207 593 2001
www.baaf.org.uk

PPIAS
(Parent to Parent Information on Adoption Services)
The Laurels
Lower Boddington
Daventry
Northants NN11 6YB
Tel: 01295 660 121
Fax: 01295 660 123

Overseas Adoption Helpline
1st Floor
34 Upper Street
London N1 0PN
Tel: 0207 226 7666

Department of Health
Community Services Division CS3B
Wellington House
133–155 Waterloo Road
London SE1 8UG
Tel: 0207 972 4084

Home Office Immigration and Nationality Department
Linar House
40 Wellesley Road
Croydon CR9 2BY
Tel: 0208 686 0688
www.perspectivespress.com

9   Fostering

People who consider **fostering** as opposed to adoption, tend to be adults with previous experience of parenting. Fostering actually means having a special non-blood-linked relationship by virtue of nursing or bringing up. The term refers to the promotion of growth of a child and the affectionate tending of a child to cherish and provide for. In today's practice, it implies 'shared parenting'. There are both short- and long-term aims associated with fostering. In the short term, fostering should provide a safe place for a child where the process of finding/providing whatever is necessary for the child in the long-term will begin.

Unlike adoption, some aspects of fostering could include **rehabilitation**, or preparation for adoption. Long-term fostering tends to be organised for older children, particularly for those who cannot go to their parental home for care, but who need to keep their family connections. Reasons why children cannot live in their parental home can be because the child behaves in a way the family cannot deal with, or because the family situation cannot provide for the child in emotional, social or any other terms. Thus fostering may be an option for infertile individuals as one means to have a child to look after, but it is not a child to keep. This may put many infertile individuals off this option, and indeed research suggests that few infertile couples considered fostering as an option to overcome their childlessness (van den Akker, 1998c). However, caring for a child and being able to meet his or her demands when he or she is happy or disturbed is one of the central tasks of parenting in any situation. If we think rationally about the needs of involuntarily childless people wishing to become a family, it is surprising that fostering is very rarely considered by the same people who believe that having children will result in a more fulfilling life. The main argument against fostering is the likely age of the child and the temporary nature of a foster family. However, repeated fostering and long-term contact is often possible, showing that perhaps the negative profile of fostering should be reconsidered.

Although the term 'fostering' is often used synonymously with 'parenting', it is also described as a 'job', or as 'employment' because fees are paid to the foster parent(s), training is provided, and a partnership with other agencies (for example, social workers, social services) is involved. Foster carers tend to be assessed and trained for their task in much the same way as adoptive parents, though of course there are also distinct differences.

Regardless of fertility status, theoretically fostering appears to be less common and perhaps even less desirable than adoption, but this may be due to inadequate knowledge about this practice. The amount of fostering literature is rapidly catching up with that of adoption, which is prolific, and much can be gained from a fair introduction to this area of child care. In 1995 Ann Wheal produced *The Foster Carer's Handbook* which deals primarily with the practicalities and responsibilities of fostering, but which also acknowledges some fundamental childrearing principles. Based on research carried out by Wheal, a list of responsibilities are seen as prerequisites for foster caring, including being aware of a child's emotional, social, educational, religious and physical needs. A list incorporating these essential carer qualities was compiled, and a summary of these is given in Box 9.1.

Box 9.1   Carer qualities needed in fostering

- Provide each child with nutrition and a personal space
- Share activities with the child
- Establish clear expectations and limits
- Discipline and reward the child as appropriate
- Talk with the child and allow visits to his or her birth family where appropriate
- Learn to understand the child
- Be responsible for the child's medical and dental care
- Be involved with the child's school activities and educational needs
- Respect the child
- Work with all concerned, including the child, to make a permanent plan for that child
- Help prepare the child for return to his/her parent(s) or for placement with relatives or friends or alternative long-term carers
- Help the child to speak up, to be heard and to be listened to

---

Clearly, these prerequisites are no different from those required of any parental figure, with the exception of the points relating to the promotion of good communication and relations between the child's original parental and social background. These are important points which are specific to the fostering situation and require a great deal of compassion and understanding to fulfil.

As with adoption, the foster child is likely to have been under considerable stress for a period of time. Stress or conflict may recur upon regular visits of the child to his or her original parents or guardians. These challenges must be met sensitively by the foster parents, and may require some training. In the UK, as in many other countries, recruitment campaigns for foster parents have increased over the years. Training, on the other hand, is a relatively new asset to agencies dealing with fostering, and this practice is still in its infancy.

There are no uniform procedures for admission of children to foster care homes. This may be because fewer foster parents make themselves available than adoptive parents. One consistent criterion looked for in prospective foster parents is that they have a 'mature capacity for parenthood' (Kline and Overstreet, 1972). Other than that, the aim in most cases is to ensure that parents have no psychopathology and have 'healthy' motives for fostering a child. However, what constitutes a healthy motive is not entirely clear. Altruism alone is an unlikely motive and perhaps not entirely believable. Interestingly, the fostering recruitment outlook appears to be one where some satisfaction, whether personal or financial, is not frowned upon, but accepted as a reasonable motive for fostering (Triseliotis et al., 1995). This, of course, is in contrast to surrogacy, where financial reward is regarded as unacceptable (Brazier, 1997).

In the past, applicants for fostering with entirely altruistic motives were considered to be the most suitable as foster parents. Triseliotis et al. (1995) describe the 'fears of baby farming (a legacy of the second part of the 19th century), which added to the discouragement of any reward reflected in the allowance'. These views have since changed. Two factors contributed to changing these views:

- fostering has become more specialist, and 'paid professionalism' for the 'job' of fostering is now the accepted policy on pay
- the 1983 adoption allowance schemes have been positively received.

Both these factors have contributed to the argument that 'love and money' *can* go together (Hill et al., 1989).

PSYCHOLOGICAL AND SOCIAL ASPECTS OF FOSTERING

Very little research has been carried out on the psychological and social aspects of fostering. Most research has drawn on the adoption literature, but that, unfortunately, does not provide valid comparisons for fostering. Fostering is almost always temporary, and foster parents often foster one child after another. Foster children tend to be moved from temporary home to temporary home, until a suitable solution to their placement problem is found. This solution may result in adoption or going back to the child's original biological environment.

Very few infertile individuals choose fostering, mainly because it is only a temporary solution to their childlessness (van den Akker, 1998c). Future research could assess the impact of fostering on foster parents and the children. Such research could inform those who know little about the practice and perhaps make it a feasible temporary option for the many infertile couples seeking to create a family. Fertile foster carers or parents tend to live happy lives, feeling able to contribute positively to a child's needs, and many foster children remain in contact with their foster parents if the environment was supportive.

The pain and separation for children and their families are characteristic pictures of foster care. It is therefore no surprise that many foster children have been reported as having problems in forming relationships (Fein, 1991). However, despite the instability in the social environment of foster children, research also documents good to adequate functioning overall in foster children (Festinger, 1983). In fact, some studies suggest that children in foster care did better on some psychological indicators than those who returned home (Wald et al., 1988). However, this tended to be the case mainly for children who had remained in relatively stable and longer-term foster care (Fanshel et al., 1989).

Most of the research carried out on foster care has come from the US. There, evidence suggests that biological parents visiting their children were more likely to be reunited (Fein et al., 1983), although this visiting of the biological parent has also been known to deteriorate the foster parent–child relationship. The focal point of fostering is the quality and stability of the foster home (parents). If fostering can be longer term, the early problems faced through separation can be overcome. Fostering has been a neglected area in research, but considering that the welfare of the child should always be first and foremost in the mind of anyone creating a family, fostering for the benefit of the child should be a rewarding form of parenting.

FURTHER INFORMATION

Further information about fostering can be obtained from the following organisations.

BAAF
(British Association for Adoption and Fostering)
Head Office
Skyline House
200 Union Street
London SE1 0LY
Tel: 0207 593 2000
Fax: 0207 593 2001
www.baaf.org.uk

National Foster Care Association
Francis House
Francis Street
London SW1P 1DE
Tel: 0208 286 266

Local Social Services

10   Issues for those Involved
       in Infertility Treatments

DONOR ISSUES

Infertility treatment would not be as advanced as it is today if it was not for the donation of genetic material by one person for use by another. Donations of sperm, egg or pre-embryo are now successful and commonplace. Medical considerations include the selection of donors, evaluation of the recipients and quality control of the genetic material (Eisenberg and Schenker, 1998). Social and psychological considerations include the resolving of conflicts, emotions and the importance or lack of importance of a genetic link. Economic considerations include the use of these services when there are many children waiting to find good homes, both in the UK and abroad; moral, legal and ethical considerations include the ownership of the genetic material and the discarding of gametes or embryos in cases of abortions, to name but a few.

Donor issues have, until recently, been relatively neglected. There are many ethical issues to be considered in donating one's own genetic material, and this practice of donation is much more common in men than women. Although it would be easy to think that men find it easier not to be emotionally involved with any possible offspring, the real reason for the difference is the tremendous amount of effort that a woman needs to expend in donation compared to a man. For a woman, donating involves the surgical collection of the eggs after prolonged drug treatment (as described in Chapter 6). The discomfort and risks involved to the woman in taking drugs to stimulate ovarian activity for egg retrieval should not be underestimated.

Donors are provided with some information to ensure that, as far as is reasonably possible, they are well informed about their decision to donate. Donors are free to withdraw their **consent** at any stage although, of course, once the gametes have been used in treatment it is too late. A woman donating eggs goes through a more expensive treatment procedure than a man donating his sperm. However, if the woman decides to withdraw her consent, even after preparations for egg recovery have started, she will not be penalised in any form, including financially. Donors are also informed that use of their gametes in treatment will stop once up to ten children have been conceived from them. They may, however, state a lower maximium number if they so wish. Donors will also be made aware of the importance of accurate information on the forms, because the consequences of completing the form inaccurately can have devastating consequences for the recipient family and the donor child. Furthermore, the consequences can also extend to themselves, because once a donor child born with a defect or disability reaches the age of 18, he or she can sue the donor if the latter failed to disclose information relating to this.

Clinics involved in providing donated gametes (sperm or eggs) for the treatment of infertility are required to go through a series of assessments and considerations of donors, as described in Box 10.1.

Box 10.1   Assessment of and information provided by donors

- Take a family history
- Take a medical history
- The presence of any heritable disorders or transmissible infection
- Level of potential fertility of semen
- Discuss the possible implications if a child born from their donation is disabled
- Discuss the number of children their donations are allowed to create
- Whether they already have their own children
- Their attitude toward donation
- Discuss issues of anonymity
- The donor's legal position needs to be made clear (HFEA *Code of Practice*, 1993)

Sperm donors currently receive £15 per donation, plus expenses for their contribution. They are assured that they will not be considered to be the legal father of any child resulting from their donation, and that they hold no parental responsibility for the child(ren). However, legally, anyone donating gametes must provide information about themselves to the HFEA, who record the information on a confidential information register. Necessary information includes name and date of birth. In addition to this, other (non-identifying) information is required, such as eye and hair colour, occupation and general interests. This information is scant, and does not allow donor offspring to discover anything personal about their genetic mother or father. Ironically, the HFEA states that when considering using treatment with donated gametes, one consideration for the couple intending to use donated gametes must be their ability to cope with any donor child(ren)'s need 'to know' about his or her origins. Donor offspring have access to this information when they reach the age of 18, or if they wish to marry someone to whom they are related, but it is clearly not enough. Box 10.2 outlines the main points of any client assessment and information.

Box 10.2   Assessment of and information provided by clients (prospective parents)

- Take a family history
- Take a medical history
- Discuss the possible implications if a child born disabled or with multiple births
- Find out about the clients' commitment to having and bringing up children
- Find out if they can provide a stable and supportive environment for the child
- Ascertain their health and ages and consequent future ability to look after a child
- Discuss the effect of a new baby on existing children in the family

---

Disclosure of donor insemination origins has also been subject to intense investigation. This is because it was known that many people did not tell their child that donor gametes were used in conception, thereby pretending they were the **genetic parents** when in fact they were not. In Sweden, the law was changed in 1985 allowing all donor insemination offspring the right to obtain **identifying information** about the donor providing the sperm for conception. The same legal changes were made in Austria in 1992 and in Victoria, Australia, in 1995. This was seen as a risky decision, because other countries argued that it would stop donors from coming forward and thus lead to a shortage of donors. Although initially this was indeed the case in Sweden, the number of prospective donors increased again sometime later, and back to the original number. Gottlieb et al. (2000) studied Swedish parents who had used donor insemination after the 1985 legislation to determine how many would tell their child that they were not genetically related. They found that the majority of parents (89%) had not informed their child(ren), and 59% had told someone else. The worry here is that these children may find out from someone else how they were conceived.

Not only should egg and sperm donors be given the opportunity to receive counselling, but the grown-up children of this technique should also be given the opportunity to receive counselling if they so wish. There may be identity problems, or a desperate wish to find out more about their donor 'parent(s)'. Crammond (1998) assessed the literature on the counselling needs of patients receiving donated gametes. The following areas were identified for counselling if the recipient couple are to cope adequately with the donation on an interpersonal level and if they are to make sense of their experience:

- concerns, feelings and attitudes towards the donor
- the role of the donor in the couple's relationship
- feelings about not being the genetic parent
- whether to disclose the donation to the potential child and others.

Research into disclosure of the genetic origins of offspring brought about through donation is also becoming increasingly important. With the increase in donation possibilities and the successes described in disclosure of adoption, legislators are increasingly concerned to follow good practice for the many millions of children born through donated sperm, eggs or gametes. A recent study investigated the reasoning behind parental disclosure of their children's genetic origins (Nachtigall et al., 1998). Nachtigall et al. found that of 70 men and 86 women who had children through donor insemination treatment, 30% said they would disclose this to their children, but a larger percentage (54%) would not, or remained undecided (16%). These numbers are somewhat surprising, because the adoption literature suggests that most adoptees wish to know about their genetic origins. If the best interests of the child are considered, clearly non-disclosing parents are not considering the child's needs, but their own. The reasoning behind the decision to tell was to be 'honest', whereas reasons not to tell were seen as '**confidentiality**' issues. Since donor children are not few and far between, but now form large populations in their own right across the world, it is time to consider the impact of being and finding out that you are a donor child. Table 10.1 gives the numbers of DI children born per year and overall in various countries, to demonstrate the popularity of this treatment.

Table 10.1   Numbers of donor insemination (DI) children born per year and total populations (if recorded)

Country	Per year	Total DI population
US	30000	1000000
Australia	2000	–
Japan	–	10000
France	1700	16000
The Netherlands	> 1000	–
Switzerland	> 1000	–
Sweden	> 300	–

Leiblum and Aviv (1998) also studied **disclosure** issues and decisions of couples who used DI. In this study 27 couples with male factor infertility completed a questionnaire concerned with disclosure issues. Nearly three-quarters had not disclosed DI to their child and had no intention of doing so in the future. However, 85% had confided to at least one other person about their DI conception. What was particularly interesting about the results of this study was that approximately one-third of the sample said that they did not know how or when to disclose this information to their child. This shows the lack of guidance available to infertile people opting for DI once conception has taken place. Most of the couples in Leiblum and Aviv's study were not offered any counselling at any stage. It is therefore not surprising that without information, many people tend to do nothing, even though this may not be in their own or their child's best interests.

Few studies have focused on the importance of a genetic/ biological link between parents and their children. In studies where this has been considered, it is clear that if a genetic link is a possibility, most people would tend to opt for that type of treatment. In one of my studies I found that in cases of surrogate arrangements, the majority of women who could use their own genetic material would choose that option, whereas those who could not provide their own egg to the surrogate for implantation said they were not overly concerned about a genetic link (van den Akker, 2001a). There appears to be a prevalence of males favouring the genetic link (73.5% males versus 48.6% females), as was found in Ravin et al.'s (1997) study of men and women from the general population. These data suggest that the future of infertility treatment must consider the relevance, opportunities and coping mechanisms of couples undergoing treatment with donated genetic material. It is possible that gut preferences have to be overruled by options, and these may need to be resolved with the assistance of appropriately qualified and experienced professionals. However, with developments in reproductive technology, even women with eggs not suitable for fertilisation may be able to use their genetic material in donated gametes in the not-so-distant future. A recent paper described the development of a method of chemically and mechanically induced membrane fusion which could be used to transfer the nucleus from the egg of an infertile woman into the cytoplasm of a donor egg (Tesarik et al., 2000), thus producing a largely genetic conception.

However, until this is a practical reality, we need to continue to take account of the literature which has unravelled numerous issues requiring further thought and investigation. This is done with only one prominent focus in mind: to help infertile couples make well-informed decisions about whether or not to use donated gametes or embryos. In 1984, Aphrodite Clamar discovered an important factor which must not be forgotten – that 'infertility as a life crisis is dealt with in a vacuum'. What this refers to is the fact that the emotional turmoil experienced during investigation and treatment precludes adequate time and resources being made available for the individuals concerned to assess the wider consequences of such treatments and their own feelings towards the child, the infertile partner who was unable to contribute a genetic link to the child, the further family, the social networks. These considerations are clearly not considered fully by many people as they embark on these treatments. Whatever route is chosen, openness appears to be the best way forward, regardless of how the child was eventually conceived. Menning (1982) discusses the moral, ethical and philosophical benefits of acceptance of donation procedures, and argues against the practice of 'pretending'. Some clinics advocate 'pretending', where the infertile partner's sperm is mixed with that of the donor, keeping a degree of uncertainty about the lineage.

Others refer to this sort of practice and non-disclosure in general as families 'living a lie'.

CHILDREN PRODUCED THROUGH ARTIFICIAL REPRODUCTIVE TECHNOLOGY

Louise Brown, now 23 years old, was the first ever child to be produced in a test tube; she is healthy and content with the origins of her conception. IVF pioneers Patrick Steptoe and Robert Edwards were responsible for her conception, her transfer into her mother's uterus and her healthy delivery. Their work at the time was highly advanced, and seen by many as within the realms of science fiction, not something that would become a relatively routine intervention for many individuals with fertility problems. Louise herself has appeared in the media relatively frequently, and comes across as a well adjusted individual with a healthy mind and body. This is important, because current techniques utilised in the procreation of children are now so much further developed from the Steptoe and Edwards days that now even relatively **unviable** material, which is not necessarily healthy, is used to form embryos which are successfully transferred into the uterus.

Very few investigations into children conceived from donated gametes have been carried out. Researchers who did reported a number of problems, including:

- feeling that they did not fit in with their families because of physical differences (Baran and Pannor, 1993)
- being aware from a relatively early age that something was not said within the family (Vercollone et al., 1997)
- learning about their conception in shocking and unexpected circumstances (Snowden et al., 1983).

However, reports of positive or neutral effects have also been forthcoming, such as:

- no altered perception of existing self-concepts following disclosure (Snowden et al., 1983; Vercollone et al., 1997)
- no significant differences in socio-emotional welfare of donor offspring (children) (Golombok et al., 1999).

There is not much available information about the offspring of donated gametes, and even less about children produced through other reproductive techniques. Of particular interest for the future are issues concerned with children conceived from sperm or eggs which would not have resulted in the creation of an embryo without medical intervention. Louise Brown was created from relatively healthy gametes. However, we know little or nothing yet about children conceived from relatively unhealthy material. In the *Human Reproduction Update* issue, entirely devoted to follow-up studies of children born as a result of reproductive assistance, the findings were reassuring: Lansac and Royere (2001) reported no difference in chromosomal abnormalities or birth defects from the general population, and no negative health in children born from frozen sperm; the general health of offspring born from oocyte donation was within normal limits (Soderstrom-Anttila, 2001); the physical, language and motor development of children up to two years old born as a result of IVF surrogacy was good (Serafini, 2001); as were the parent–child relationships between donor insemination children and their parents (Braeways, 2001). As a result of confidentiality regulations, it is difficult to access information on such children's psychosocial development. However, some researchers managed to study oocyte donor offspring up to the age of eight years, and their psychosocial functioning was also reported to be healthy (Applegarth et al., 1995; Soderstrom-Anttila et al., 1998).

Alexina McWhinnie confirms some of the problems parents of donor offspring have. She studied 31 families with children born following IVF and ICSI, and compared them to children born after donor insemination. She found that not one single parent using donor insemination had disclosed this to the child. She found that although these parents found deceiving the child easy while the child was young, when he or she became older the parents often ran into difficulties. Offspring who found out later that their parents had kept half of their genetic identity a secret were often very angry. We know from donor offspring support groups in Australia that grown-up children conceived through donor insemination wish to know who the donors were (Dudley and Neave, 1997). Research into adoption has also demonstrated that 'open' adoption works far better than 'closed' adoption (Sants, 1964; Triseliotis, 1973; Brodzinski et al., 1992). Furthermore, individuals who find out later on in life that they are not the genetic children of the people they believed to be their parents all their lives are far more upset by this (Turner and Coyle, 2000) than individuals who have always known they were adopted or conceived with donated gametes. Openness is therefore preferable to living a life of secrecy. Daniels and Taylor (1993) asked donors if they would be happy to have identifying information about them provided to any possible children conceived as a result of their donation(s). They found that considerably more donors were happy with the possibility that their offspring would attempt to contact them in later life than is generally assumed.

PSYCHOLOGICAL INTERACTIONS WITH CHILDREN BORN THROUGH ARTIFICIAL REPRODUCTIVE TECHNOLOGY

Psychological research on infertility tends to acknowledge that the shock of the diagnosis and the stress of the treatment may have an impact on the individuals concerned. It is therefore not surprising that researchers have felt the need to investigate the psychological adaptation to any subsequent pregnancy and motherhood. A limited amount of research is available on the effects of infertility or treatment on subsequent childrearing and/or psychological effects on the child. However, those studies which have been carried out shed some light on mother–child interactions and the child's functioning.

Halman et al. (1995) studied the effects of infertility on adaptation to pregnancy and early motherhood. They found little to worry about, with previously infertile women adapting well to their pregnancy and identifying well with their role as a mother. Previously infertile women were also slightly more in control of their labour and delivery than their comparison group of fertile women. A Dutch investigator (van Balen, 1996) studied over 100 parents of two- to four-year-old children. His study groups consisted of parents who conceived by IVF, parents who were previously infertile and parents who were fertile. He found that a greater amount of emotional involvement with the child was reported in IVF and previously infertile mothers compared to fertile mothers. Parental competence was also higher in the infertile and IVF groups, and these same groups rated their children more often as social and less often as obstinate than the fertile mothers. Interestingly, no significant group or fertility status differences were observed in the three groups of fathers.

In the US, Allen et al. (1996) reported on 45 women with a history of infertility and compared these with 45 fertile women who had **delayed childbearing**. Previously infertile women were no more likely to experience adjustment difficulties in dealing with their children, to experience feelings of isolation or to feel restricted and unsupported than the fertile delayed childbearing group. In summary, pregnancy following treatment for infertility is recognised as a major life event. The consequences of the diagnosis and treatment tend to have no adverse effects on the previously infertile couple's ability to deal with the pregnancy, delivery and subsequent childrearing.

WHEN THINGS GO WRONG

In any one year some mistakes are made, and a fraction of these reach us, the public, through the media. For example, one recent high-profile case concerned a private London clinic which was sued successfully by a man for using his frozen sperm for insemination into his ex-girlfriend. He had not wanted to have a child with this woman, and he had not been aware that his own gametes were being used without his consent. This is just one case, but consider what the implications of such occurrences are. First, there is now a child whose father will not recognise her. At some time she will probably discover that her mother used illegal means to obtain the sperm, and that the clinic was not authorised to use it in IVF treatment. We do not know what the likely effects might be on the child, but we do know that the creation of this child is a far cry from creating a child through desire and altruism on the donor's part.

Another example of the opportunity for malpractice comes from further abroad. Two well known Israeli infertility specialists were investigated for claims that they sold other women's ova on the 'black market'. Their crime lay in their excessive overstimulation of ovaries of patients undergoing ovarian harvesting in order to produce as many ova as they could, and them selling the surplus to infertile women in Israel and abroad. Apart from the risks this creates for the targeted women undergoing this not very pleasant procedure, those same women also now have to live with the knowledge that some of their ova were successfully utilised in IVF with other patients. Consequently, their child(ren) may be cared for by other 'parents', not by themselves. This may be even more devastating if they have themselves had IVF failures.

These are not isolated cases of mistakes or malpractice and there are other ways to focus our thoughts on whether or not we are doing the right thing. Consider, for example, a recent one-day conference in London which focused on the welfare of the child. At this conference, the director of the Multiple Births Foundation, Jane Denton, said that much more research effort should go into the welfare of the children produced as the result of infertility treatment. She pointed out that the social and economic effects of multiple births, a common occurrence in fertility treatment, will have implications for the family and the children. Meeting the children's requirements means the sharing of time and resources between all of them; the parents may not be able to cope with the demands of two, three or more children, and the financial burden can be catastrophic.

These utterly practical and common-sense warnings were contrasted with the chances of success at conception. Hossam Abdalla pointed out that, unfortunately, whether or not the burden of multiple births is great, it may be less of a disadvantage than not having conceived at all. Since the success rates increase with the transfer of three embryos compared to two or one, it would be disastrous for many couples if legislation insisted on a low number of transfers. Here, the social, economic and clinical perspectives provide the same issues in a different light. Who is to decide what is right and wrong and how do we determine whether social and/or economic factors should override clinical ones, or vice versa? What is probably important to remember is that any undertaking carries with it risks. The alternative is to do nothing. If, on the other hand, any action is taken when the person is armed with excellent knowledge of the costs and benefits involved, then the impact of risk can be taken responsibly.

Other problems include what to do with shared embryos in cases of separation or divorce of the prospective parents, being prepared for a multiple pregnancy and the subsequent delivery and care of the babies; foetal reduction; foetal reduction and miscarriage; running out of time, money, physical or psychological resources to continue; and, finally, failure to conceive following years of trying. The giving up part can be as difficult as the diagnosis part at the start of the enquiries in infertility.

GIVING UP TREATMENT

Women's feelings about involuntary childlessness following abandonment of treatment have been investigated by Daniluk (1996). She found that during the treatment phase, women were hopeful about conception and did not consider themselves as biologically childless, but as 'not yet pregnant'. It was only once they had taken the decision to abandon treatment totally that they came to terms with the reality of their situation. In other words, they began the slow and 'painful process of letting go of their hopes and dreams, and of coming to terms with the fact that they would never likely bear a child'.

In studying people who give up treatment, research has concentrated on those who have tried and failed. We already know from earlier in the book that each clinic has a duty to make it clear to their patients what the success rates of the treatment are. We also know that success can be achieved in different ways, and that overall it is not successful for many people. Thus, although many patients receiving treatment are aware of this fact, when attempts at treatment fail the consequences can be devastating. Trounson and Wood (1981) reported marked increases in depression in failed embryo transfers and IVF treatments. Alternatively, infertile people seeking treatment may be rejected for medical or psychological and social grounds, as pointed out by Edelmann (1990). Edelmann reviewed some of the issues involved in patient selection or assessment in psychological terms. He, and others (Greenfield and Haseltine, 1986), note that it is extremely difficult to decide on who should assess patients for suitability, what should be used to determine suitability and when suitability assessments should best be carried out. Even if an optimum professional measure and time is found, it is possible that infertile populations will respond with bias, knowing that a good profile is more likely to get them accepted than an unstable profile.

Edelmann's review of the literature shows that studies monitoring patients following a failed first IVF cycle reported that 21% of patients whose first treatment failed opted for counselling (Greenfield et al., 1988). Grief scores were higher in women who **discontinued treatment** at mid-cycle (Reading, 1989) and feelings of sadness and depression were higher in women failing to conceive following treatment (Leiblum et al., 1987; Baram et al., 1988).

If a decision is to be made about abandoning all hope of ever having a baby, some support will be necessary. A couple deciding to stop trying, whether a joint decision or a unilateral one, need to be able to cope with the decision. If a unilateral decision is made, a great rift is likely to appear between the partners. Where a mutual decision is made, it is probably still beneficial to talk this over with others. The British Organisation of Non-Parents could be a useful source.

COUNSELLING

Counselling has been mentioned several times so far in this book, but because it often has a major role to play in good outcome, adjustment and further psychosocial functioning, it deserves a section to itself. Another reason to consider counselling separately is because the choices are numerous, provided the infertility condition, the availability of resources and the costs allow it. Counselling, in essence, involves the patient requesting or being offered some form of help in addition to the physical and technological care given as part of the treatment. Alternatively, a GP or specialist may suggest that the patient would benefit from counselling. Counselling is built upon a relationship between the patient(s) and the counsellor, who can be seen as a facilitator to help bring about change in the person. Furthermore, the HFEA states clearly that all clinics offering fertility treatment must make counselling available. Although the offer of counselling is a condition of holding a licence for the treatment centre, it is not compulsory for the client or patient to take it up. It should therefore be available if the individual or couple thinks it will be of benefit to them. (A detailed historical account of the HFEA's involvement with counselling in infertility treatment is provided in an excellent book devoted to infertility counselling by Jennings, 1995.)

There are three broad categories of counselling which may be needed in infertility investigations or treatment.

- **Implications counselling**. Here the implications of diagnosis or treatment are discussed. The focus is not just on the individual, but extends to the concerns of other relatives, any existing children or those born as the result of treatment, and the wider social environment. Also included in implications counselling is genetic counselling, if appropriate. A number of specific issues need to be part of the process of implications counselling in infertility treatment centres, particularly if donated eggs or sperm are used. The HFEA has made it clear that individuals undergoing treatment with donated material ought to be aware of the social responsibilities incurred, what the effects of the 'revolutionary' procedures will be and how they may feel about discarding any spare embryos or gametes
- **Supportive counselling**. As the term suggests, this is used primarily to support the individual with specific issues or problems, or with the stress of the decision-making or treatment experienced. Supportive counselling can take place prior to, during or following treatment, particularly if no pregnancy has been established. Many adjustments may have

to be made because one or more options initially chosen may turn out to be inappropriate, or may even fail. Supportive counselling can assist someone in coming to terms with this and may help in the cognitive restructuring which may be necessary in the consideration of future alternative options or giving up treatment

- **Therapeutic counselling**. The aim of this is to therapeutically assist the individual in coping with the investigations and treatments. This tends to be an ongoing process in which the counsellor attempts to help the individual to accept or to adjust to their particular situation.

The amount of counselling needed, as with the type of counselling needed, depends entirely on the individual's circumstances and perceived needs. There are no hard-and-fast rules, and anyone can start or terminate the counselling provided as and when he or she wishes. Of course, in some situations the counsellor will be able to advise a particular course of action to help the individual obtain the optimum benefit of the sessions.

Counsellors may be most effective if they work as part of the clinic's team. Fortunately, in some clinics this is the case, and counsellors are deeply involved with the procedures, the individuals concerned and the team and its workings. There are many more clinics, however, that are not as fortunate as this. In these cases, a counsellor is contracted to come in for appointments with individuals, or individuals may be provided with a list of a few counsellors in their local area. This is generally less satisfactory, because not all 'outside' counsellors will have regular contact with individuals with fertility problems, and even less will have a deep knowledge and experience of the more revolutionary techniques practised.

Researchers have pointed out there is to date no systematic assessment of the impact of infertility, and no one knows what the most effective form of psychological counselling is. In the 1980s, Edelmann and Connolly (1986) described the state of the counselling literature as exceedingly limited, as little research evidence has been used to evaluate the problems faced. Today, not much appears to have changed. We still do not know what the needs of infertile couples are, we do not know what coping strategies they use, and we do not know what success in counselling means. However, we do know that not all the patients' needs are met.

Two studies of patient satisfaction have revealed that counselling or support, particularly *after* treatment, is seen as beneficial (Donegan, 1994; Smith et al., 2000). In Donegan's study, satisfaction with care decreased markedly following treatment failure, whereas in Smith et al.'s study unrealistic expectations were prevalent despite adequate information. This study showed that some form of information-based emotional care should be provided at all stages of the treatment process. As many treatments are carried out in NHS-funded clinics, that do not necessarily have counselling staff as part of the in-house team, inappropriate choices, from an emotional perspective regarding the outcome of treatment option chosen and lack of support to help couples cope with decisions, could be avoided using appropriately trained and informed counsellors.

Schmidt (1998) used a **grounded theory** approach to analyse the information obtained from infertile couples themselves (a rare type of study in infertility research) about how they assessed their infertility treatment and what they saw as their needs. Interesting results were obtained, ranging from a preference for specialist small clinics, with fewer staff and shorter waiting times, to following a treatment plan known to both the doctor and the patient. Surprisingly, the patients' assessment of treatment was not at all related to outcome or type of treatment received, but in general a great deal of dissatisfaction with the lack of emotional care was expressed. Schmidt concluded that the health care system fails to meet the many needs of infertile couples, including information needs, psychological needs and sexual counselling needs. This need for and consistent lack of inclusion of counselling in the clinical management of infertility is further demonstrated by Wingfield et al. (1997). These authors set up an endometriosis clinic as a co-operative between the gynaecologists involved and a self-help group. The major source of satisfaction came from the opportunity of having consultations with a counsellor (97%). The benefits of counselling are therefore repeatedly indicated in current research, even though the process needs have not yet been fully evaluated.

Other problems with evaluating the effectiveness or otherwise of counselling provision and content concerns the fact that few infertile individuals or couples accept the offer of counselling. What is it about those who accept counselling which is different from those who do not accept counselling? It is possible that many people adjust well and do not feel the need for counselling; alternatively, counselling may be seen as threatening. Some studies have shown that even if counselling is made available, not all patients want to take up the opportunity (Shaw et al., 1988; van den Akker, 1999).

Counselling has been reported as effective in dealing with reactions to infertility (Rosenfeld and Mitchell, 1979). Social work resources might also be helpful (Houghton, 1984), and there may be a role for clinical psychologists (Humphrey, 1984). However, until research has determined what the needs are, how they are best addressed and what constitutes good outcome, it is probably best to assume that the help currently offered is more likely to be beneficial rather than harmful. It is hoped that in the future, counselling, whoever provides it, can become more specific and more effective.

FURTHER INFORMATION

Further information on donors can be obtained from the following organisations.

NEEDS
(National Egg and Embryo Donation Society)
Department of Reproductive Medicine
Regional IVF Unit
St Mary's Hospital
Whitworth Park
Manchester M13 0JH
Tel: 0161 276 6000
Fax: 0161 224 0957

DI Network
PO Box 265
Sheffield S3 7YX
0114 245 4369
www.Issue.co.uk/dinet/

Further details of counselling services are available from the following organisations.

Family Care
21 Castle Street
Edinburgh EH2 3DN
Tel: 0131 225 6441

Infertility Support Group
c/o Women's Health and Reproductive Rights
Information Centre
52–54 Featherstone Street
London EC1Y 8RT
Tel: 0207 251 6580

CHILD
Charter House
3 St Leonards Road
Bexhill on Sea
East Sussex TN40 1JA
Tel: 01424 732 361
Fax: 01424 731 858
www.child.org.uk/

Foresight:
Association for the Promotion of Preconceptual Care
The Old Vicarage
Church Lane
Witley
Godalming
Surrey GU8 5PN
Tel: 012879 4500

NORCAP
(National Association for Counselling Adoptees and Parents)
3 New High Street
Headington
Oxford OX3 7AJ
Tel: 01865 750 554

11   Ethical Issues

Reproductive techniques can only be made public if and when society accepts them as uncontroversial and non-threatening. If a particular technique is considered controversial, it can and will be condemned by those against the practices concerned. Controversy and condemnation tend to be founded on ethical and moral considerations. **Ethical** issues are important considerations in human reproduction. They refer to aspects of moral conduct and fair, considerate, non-threatening means and procedures to achieve a positive outcome for all concerned with reproductive interventions. These interventions range from donor issues to the use of frozen gametes; positive outcome refers to the resultant offspring and the 'others' or adults involved in the reproductive process (including donors, recipients and professional staff). Ethical issues relating to the procedures involved include issues of threat to the treated individual's health, the health and social burden of multiple pregnancies, **embryo reduction** techniques and novel means of separating embryos and implanting these at different times in the recipient. Recent advances in screening embryos for fatal chromosomal defects so that only non-defective embryos are transferred, thereby minimising the chances of failed pregnancies; rationing of services, purchasing of services and other economic factors associated with assisted fertilisation and embryo research all need to be addressed.

Morality, or moral principles, follow, to some extent, certain points of ethics. A moral is concerned particularly with the goodness or badness of some issue under consideration with the distinction between right and wrong; with virtue. Considerations of moral issues cover the moral status of gametes, the egg, the sperm and the fertilised egg. Individuals have to consider the moral constraints on trying artificial reproductive technology (ART) at any cost, or where limits might be crossed. Can some of the procedures be considered dehumanising rather than human-needs enhancing? And what are the social implications of the widespread use of ART? These moral questions can be looked at from numerous perspectives (see Box 11.1).

Box 11.1 Moral perspectives

Moral considerations of the procedures

- Freedom of choice
- Unnatural process
- Designer pregnancies/babies
- A medical/technological event

Moral considerations

- The gametes, sperm and egg independently
- The zygote, fused egg and sperm prior to implantation
- The frozen fertilised eggs
- The implanted zygote
- Donated gametes
- Donated embryos
- Sex selection
- Surrogate motherhood

- The leftover embryo frozen, immortal
- The lack of regulated oversight of the stored material
- The combination of millions of stored embryos
- Cloning
- Who has parental rights
- Pregnancies in older women
- Genetic screening for 'defects'
- Selective abortion of multiple foetuses

Moral implications of widespread ART use

- Artificially created shift in balance between male/female ratio
- Possible homogeneity of society

- Possible decline of the traditional two-parent heterosexual family
- Possible unknown relatedness of individuals created through ART

In any discussion of morals or ethics, particularly in relation to the medical profession's move from treating illness to intervening to bring something about, there is a need for some critical reflection of the traditional norms governing the **therapeutic** relationship to 'do no harm'. The medical professional's obligation to 'do no harm' is based not only on a negative duty of non-maleficence, but also on a positive duty of beneficence. This is an aspect of the trusting relationship between the clinician and the patient. Until roughly 50 years ago, for example, family planning or contraception was often condemned as an immoral practice, making access to such 'intervention' difficult, particularly for the financially or educationally disadvantaged of the population. Since the 1960s human rights issues and understanding have made access to fertility care (contraception, abortion and fertility treatment) easier. Despite this, the 'rights' issue in human rights has now become more rather than less complicated, because we need to disentangle the consensus of the balance of rights for the 'mother' and the 'father', and the foetus, embryo or gamete. Attempts are now being made to draw the population more deeply into the debates by making more information accessible to those using fertility interventions and those not using it. The WHO has provided an electronic link or review library which gives information about reproductive decision-making in health issues, particularly in developing countries (Major, 2000). **Public debate** can inform and clarify the difficult decisions which may have to be made in reproductive health. Some insight into the consequences of reproductive technology is essential, particularly if this is done reflectively.

Holloway (1999) describes the pluralistic UK society which holds within it many different value systems. He describes the value systems of some people as the 'passive logic' of those who, to put it simply, see nature as fixed and unalterable, and others whose value systems permit interventions into the processes of nature. The latter place a veto on any procedures which could artificially interfere with the creation of life itself. A third category of value systems described by Holloway adopts a developmental approach to intervening with nature. He describes it as 'the result of the application of human consciousness to the universe itself'. This approach accepts the human spirit of enquiry against a backdrop of caution to do no harm. In countries where regulation has been implemented for various techniques, the intention is to accept rather than ban certain methods.

However, there is more at stake here than the debating of individual techniques. Each and every development is likely to have direct or indirect spin-offs. The rapid breakthroughs in human reproductive technology have provided a means of studying ovulation, fertilisation and the early stages of human embryonic development. This has resulted in knowledge about events taking place in the very first days of life which programme subsequent foetal development and which influence the pattern of disease in later life. Such new knowledge is beneficial in terms of prevention of disease and under-standing the course of disease from inception. Huge sections of the population are therefore in favour of embryonic research, but there are also many against it. This requires a fine balance in regulations and legislation. The **pre-embryo** can be seen as no more than a cluster of cells, and it has been argued that this should not be considered any different from any other tissue culture examined and manipulated under the microscope. Others believe that embryos are human beings, have parents and can be orphaned and murdered. Either way, although there seems to be a gradual acceptance of fertility treatments, this acceptance is accompanied by increasing fears that these processes might get out of hand.

For example, historical differences in cultural attitudes and beliefs to donation will affect individuals differently. Many traditional religions, such as Roman Catholicism, see the use of donor insem-ination as akin to adultery involving unacceptable practices such as masturbation, and see it as morally repugnant (although they accept other methods to achieve the collection of sperm). Islam and Judaism also find DI objectionable, but base their objections on a different principle, objecting to the loss of identifiable lineage and the dangers of future incestuous marriages. Israel is in fact on the verge of passing a new parliamentary bill to allow Israeli women to donate their eggs to other Israeli women. The recommendations have been endorsed by leading rabbis. The bill is based on highly detailed recommendations safeguarding against mixing of religions, future incestuous marriages, and making provisions for anonymity and compensation for the donor's time, loss of income and discomfort (Siegel-Itzkovich, 2001).

Religious and non-religious groups and individuals are having to interpret the moral acceptability of each new technique as it is made available. Ironically, some may object to the experimentation and development of new techniques yet accept the outcome of those developments. For most people, in theory the idea of donation of blood, organs, sperm or eggs is seen as morally acceptable if it is based on the principles of altruism. If it is seen as a commercial venture, more objections are voiced. Yet in practice, men tend to be more likely to donate if they get paid for it, whereas women tend to donate for altruistic reasons (in any case they are *not* paid for their donation). So the entire issue is muddled by inconsistencies in views versus actions of those actually involved in donating their gametes.

Further ethical dilemmas arise which we have to consider. For example, anonymity, the selection of donors, treatment of single women, selection of recipients on social and medical grounds, sex selection and the child's right to know his or her origins. Twins and higher multiple births tend to be at a disadvantage from the start and may suffer short- and long-term consequences of their prematurity and intrauterine growth retardation. Disability is common, and if a co-twin is healthy, he or she may suffer as a result from a disabled or deceased twin. Even if co-twins are healthy, documentation exists to suggest that their development may be impaired as a result of their simultaneous demands for attention and stimulation (Bryan, 1992). Other behavioural problems are also common in multiple-birth children, and mothers commonly tend to be depressed (Botting et al., 1990). One solution currently practised is embryo reduction. Here one or more embryos are chosen to die through medical intervention, to increase the chances of survival of the others in multiple pregnancies. Alternatively, as most professional societies have issued guidelines to diminish the number of embryos to be transferred, the unacceptably high incidence of multiple pregnancies as a consequence of ART should become a thing of the past. Unfortunately, the incidence of multiple pregnancies remains high due to the pressure put on clinics to increase overall success rates. One solution proposed by Pennings (2000) is to put the moral onus on the practising physicians by extending their responsibilities from ART to the pregnancy, delivery and neonatal care of their patients.

Although most reproductive techniques are now routine, there are ethical factors to be considered because of the lack of long-term follow-up data. We do not know what effects low-quality spermatozoa chosen for injection have; we do not know anything about the consequences of using the injection of paternal **mitochondrial** DNA, asynchrony between cell cycles of the oocyte and the spermatozoon, **incomplete genomic imprinting** of both gametes, or the chromosomal consequences of incomplete oocyte activation. Treating patients with known conditions is also an issue currently being addressed. For example, most clinics will refuse to provide infertility treatment to individuals with an assumed risk of viral transmission of a disease, or with an assumed concern for their life expectancy, as in patients with HIV. A recent *BMJ* editorial (Gilling-Smith et al., 2001) suggests it is time to provide treatment for infertility to HIV-positive patients, as there is no ethical justification for withholding treatment from such patients.

The HFEA reported in 1996 that as many as 666 oocytes were donated compared to only 104 embryos. Although there is some research on oocyte donors, little is known about people donating embryos. This is because there is a lack of input from qualified academic psychologists and other scientists in this area. Research evidence of good or poor practice or good or poor outcome can assist in ethical decision-making. Other arguments drifting through the ethical dilemmas in fertility treatment surround different angles of **quality-of-life** issues. For example, when we talk about quality of life, or frustration in life, we could look at the individual wanting to have a child. If such an individual believes having a child would greatly enhance his or her life, then his or her quality of life could be improved through fertility interventions. If we look at it from the point of view of the resultant child, who is to say that the child's being has added quality of life to its existence? One could argue that maximising numbers of lives improves their quality, but then why is abortion also funded? The argument is that funding needs to be considered across the board in reproductive care, including antenatal and gynaecological care, abortions, the cost of special care babies (prevalent in multiple pregnancies, which in turn are prevalent in assisted reproduction), and so on.

Funding issues extend beyond the immediate what, who and where questions. Is the population as a whole happy with the private versus NHS funding options, and with regional variations in funding (the so-called postcode lottery) and differences in ethnicity in use of services? Overall, the current mix of public and private funding sources is inefficient and inequitable, and adequate primary prevention strategies are not initiated. Since resources are limited, professionals need to choose between competing couples in an attempt to 'maximise the number of happy children made per pound spent' (Lockwood, 1996). The consequences of the chosen technique, also called 'rationing', lead inevitably to unjustifiable and unacceptable discrimination against those who are less affluent, less articulate or older.

An ethical choice cannot be made in isolation from the feasible alternatives. Templeton (1996) reported on a large study using 36,961 cycles in the analyses and found that the predicted live birth rate per cycle started for women aged 25 was 16.1%, whilst for those aged 45 years it was a meagre 1.9%. Furthermore, at each age group over 30, donor eggs resulted in a significantly higher pregnancy rate than own-egg treatments. This has ethical dilemmas for the infertile: they may achieve a much-wanted pregnancy relatively easily using donated eggs but have a partially non-genetic child, or they may have great difficulty in conceiving using their own gametes, with a less likely success rate and hence less chance of conceiving a genetically related child (see Figure 11.1).

Other spin-offs of reproductive experimentation include **DNA** mapping, **isolating genes** and storing genes, as these are accompanied by techniques to modify or transform them. **Pre-conception** and **prenatal** screening and testing function in part to inform those involved of the condition of the likely offspring. This is generally considered morally good. However, is the often covert assumption to destroy 'imperfect' embryos good? This needs to be considered carefully, because disability has been described as a culturally constructed concept. Is able-bodied better than disabled? If a couple with hearing impairment would like to utilise genetic screening to determine hearing status in the embryo, is this good or bad? What if they prefer to have offspring with the disability to fit their circumstances, is that as good as a hearing-unimpaired couple preferring to have a hearing child? Lawson (2001) surveyed 165 women on their perceptions of raising a child with a serious disability and their attitudes towards prenatal diagnostic testing (PDT). Most women had negative views of raising a child with a disability. Women were most likely to opt for PTD if they believed parenting a disabled child would not be as rewarding as parenting a healthy child.

Similar arguments hold for foetal reduction in multiple pregnancies. First-trimester foetal reduction is considered a relatively safe and

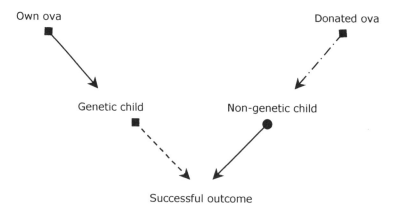

Figure 11.1   Ethical dilemmas of ART choice in relation to probabilities of success

effective option. It is effective in that it increases the prospects for the remaining embryo(s), miscarriage rates are not considered too high and it is a cost-effective technique. The reason why this technique is used is because multiple pregnancies have a higher likelihood of obstetric and perinatal morbidity and mortality. Data suggests that approximately 15% of newborn babies from multiple pregnancies do not survive beyond infancy, and a further 20% show long-term problems (Hobbins, 1988). Considering these statistics, foetal reduction is considered to be a 'rescue' technique. In psychological terms, no research to date has investigated the moral, social and psychological implications of this technique on the pregnant mothers. This is an omission which takes on a particularly sinister dimension if the pregnancy fails altogether following foetal reduction.

Thus, ethical issues are rampant throughout the area of reproductive health, functioning and treatment. Each technique carries with it some ethical issues – either directly or indirectly. Furthermore, each type of intervention has ethical similarities with others, indicating that many issues need to be addressed simultaneously by anyone involved with artificial reproductive technology. Ethics is interesting and relevant to all that we do, and I suggest that anyone involved with ART continues to read up on ethical issues, so that they have a greater understanding of the moral and ethical implications of these techniques. This is with a view to their own understanding, that of those around them, any children produced as a result of ART and the children of the future. Where do we draw the line? Is it with our own immediate needs, or is it worth considering the wider and as yet unknown implications?

FURTHER INFORMATION

For more information on ethical issues, see Lawrence Hinman, *Contemporary Moral Issues* (New Jersey: Prentice Hall, 1999). The following organisations may also provide information on ethical issues.

Enhancement Technologies Group
www.gene.ucl.ac.uk/bioethics/index.html

Euroethics
www.gwdg.de/~uelsner/euroeth.htm

World Health Organization
http://www.who.org

12   Research

No book on infertility, diagnosis or conditions requiring some form of intervention would be complete without a note on **research**. Most of what this book is based upon is research. Research means the careful search or inquiry into a particular issue deemed worthy of investigation. It uses systematic methods (of which there are many) to discover or collect facts, following a course or system of critical investigation. Many individuals seeking a diagnosis, treatment or just help and advice may find they are asked to take part in research studies or investigations. This usually means that the research participant is one of many such individuals approached for study, not that one has been carefully and selectively picked from a number. Most research is anonymous and totally confidential. In fact, from the participant's point of view (the person agreeing to take part in research) you may not even know what treatment you are receiving (although you should know you are taking part).

All research needs to be carried out by experienced researchers, taking care to follow carefully screened protocols. Most research using human participants must pass through ethical committee approval. These committees scrutinise research proposals and take special care to ensure that this type of study is ethically acceptable, will not harm the participant(s), and is feasible, justifiable and necessary. For research using gametes or embryos, researchers must apply to the HFEA for a special research licence. A licence for such research is different from human participation research. In gamete or embryo research the researchers can obtain a licence only if they can demonstrate, amongst other things, that:

- they intend to promote advances in the treatment of infertility
- they intend to increase knowledge about the early causes of congenital diseases
- they intend to increase our understanding of the causes of miscarriages.

Human participants who are able to consent to their participation in research will only be approached by a researcher or research team

despite being protected, has been challenged over time, resulting in modifications or total abandonment of earlier traditions, sometimes invariably creating new traditions in the process. Challenges to tradition invariably lead to the isolation of those challenging it – some becoming casualties (for example, Kim Cotton during the 1980s); others gaining acceptance (for example, Louise Brown as a healthy bouncy baby conceived in a test tube, or the more recent public pronouncement of gay couples becoming adoptive parents). Challenging tradition is not necessarily a disintegrating process – it can be an adaptive process. With changes to 'the way things were' one adopts new forms of being. When Edwards and Steptoe carried out their experimental test-tube baby work in the earlier part of the 1980s, the response was overtly hostile (Edwards, 1989). By 1989, IVF had become accepted as more or less mainstream. Those seeing the frighteningly rapid advances in reproductive technology and the prolific social restructuring of families may wonder what sort of society they will be living in in ten years' time. Standing still does not appeal to most individuals, so who should decide which areas should be developed further or which should be challenged and which should not?

An attitude survey carried out some ten years after the first test-tube baby demonstrated a very slow shift in the public's acceptance of the creation of alternative families if they had to make a choice. This study, on the attitudes expressed by fertile and infertile couples regarding eleven possible interventions to overcome childlessness, was carried out in 1992 by Halman et al. They questioned over 275 couples (185 were diagnosed with infertility, 90 were fertile). In 1992 some of the methods discussed in this book were not yet available in clinics. Nevertheless, the treatments used in this attitude survey covered areas where no, some or a full genetic link was present. The eleven options were: where no genetic link is present (adoption), where one of a couple maintains a genetic link (DI, artificial insemination where donor and husband's sperm are mixed, and genetic surrogacy), and where both have a genetic link (male hormonal treatment, AIH, female hormone treatment (of which there are two types), tying the cervix, IVF and gestational surrogacy). Seven options were seen favourably and four negatively by both fertile and infertile couples. Infertile couples were generally more favourable towards all interventions apart from adoption. A preference was expressed for interventions where both partners could maintain a genetic link. These results have some implications for the future of reproductive technology. The science and technology are available to provide people with a child. However, the people themselves may not be ready to accept some alternative forms of conception. This appears to be based not on the nature of the technique, but on the preference for a genetic link and on a desire for equity in the genetic link with a partner in a child. The results also shed some light on population attitudes to infertility treatments. The fertile couples responded similarly, but not as favourably to the interventions. It is likely that when couples are confronted with information, and when this is more relevant to them, their attitudes become more positive.

In short, it seems that in theory we have some ideas about and attitudes toward artificial reproductive technology, but in practice only people faced with choosing between the options available to overcome childlessness develop the knowledge needed to deal with the choice. We are endowed with a thirst for knowledge; ignorance leads to uncertainty. However, with some consensus on the benefits of progress, intelligent progress is desirable if it is adaptable. If it is adaptable, it will be sustainable. Furthermore, in terms of the future, if challenge to tradition is possible at one point, it will be so again in the future, although we may never revert back to the way things were (which is probably not a bad thing).

There are other fears apparent when we look at the future of reproductive technologies in particular. Technically we are in a position to choose the sex of a baby and to eliminate embryos with genetic diseases, and we could even be in a position to do away with reproduction altogether as it is and opt instead for cloning. European Union institutions are divided on therapeutic cloning (Watson, 2000). For example, the Netherlands has banned it (Sheldon, 2000) whereas Britain approved it initially (Fazal, 2000), and is now banning it. Other countries, such as the US, have bred babies specifically to provide stem cells for a sibling (Josefson, 2000). However, the more sophisticated the technique, the more costly it is in financial, social, psychological, moral and ethical terms. Any decisions we make now, we make for future generations. Are our desires and needs – for example, the desire for a baby – perceived as the same needs by our offspring? Is it possible that they will question our motives as being at the expense of theirs, if they had been able to have a say in it? Are we actually improving the world, or destroying something? Recent laboratory methods bridging the gap between genetically modified mice and humans have proved a 'success' in technological terms. However, the genetically modified rhesus monkey in question (ANDi) probably would not have wished to be modified with a green fluorescent protein marker, which was first isolated from glowing jellyfish and subsequently inserted into ANDi's mother's egg (Berger, 2001).

In conclusion, it is hoped that this book will have provided you, the reader, with a wide overview of infertility as it is dealt with today. The population, technological, medical, social, cultural, psychological, moral and ethical perspectives have been outlined in as concise a way as possible, without compromising the information within each chapter. The future of reproductive health and infertility in particular rests with our interpretation of the benefits and pitfalls of the past and present. One thing is for sure – without information no adequate constructs can be made and no discussions can take place.

14   Self-Help Groups

NEEDS
(National Egg and Embryo Donation Society)
Department of Reproductive Medicine
Regional IVF Unit
St Mary's Hospital
Whitworth Park
Manchester M13 0JH
Tel: 0161 276 6000
Fax: 0161 224 0957

DI Network
PO Box 265
Sheffield S3 7YX
Tel: 0114 245 4369
www.Issue.co.uk/dinet/

Infertility Support Group
c/o Women's Health and Reproductive Rights
Information Centre
52–54 Featherstone Street
London EC1Y 8RT
Tel: 0207 251 6580

ISSUE
114 Lichfield Street
Walsall WS1 1SZ
Tel: 01922 722888
Fax: 01922 640070
www.issue.co.uk

TAMBA
(Twins and Multiple Births Association)
PO Box 30
Little Sutton
South Wirral
Liverpool L66 1TH
Tel: 0151 348 0020

Tavistock Marital Studies Institute
Tavistock Centre
120 Belsize Lane
London NW3 5BA
Tel: 0121 435 7111
Fax: 0207 435 1080
www.tmsi.org.uk

15   Information Centres/Helplines

NIAC
(National Infertility Awareness Campaign)
PO Box 2106
London WIA 3D2
Tel: 0207 439 3067
www.repromed.co.uk/NIAC/info/

CHILD
Charter House
43 St Leonard's Road
Bexhill-on-Sea
East Sussex TN40 1JA
Tel: 0142 473 2361

BICA
(British Infertility Counselling Association)
Tel: 01342 843 880
www.bica.net

British Pregnancy Advisory service
Austy Manor
Wooten Wawen
Solihull
West Midlands B95 6BX
BPAS Action Line: 08457 304030
www.bpas.org

Family Planning Association
2–12 Pentonville Road
London N1 9FP
Tel: 0207 837 5432
Fax: 0207 837 3042
www.fpa.org.uk

ISSUE
114 Lichfield Street
Walsall WS1 1SZ
Tel: 01922 722888

PROGRESS
27–35 Mortimer Street
London W1N 7RJ
Tel: 0207 436 4528

Women's Health
D.E. Tucker MRCOG
52 Featherstone Street
London EC1Y 8RT
Tel: 070 69 950 121
www.womens-health.co.uk

Children's legal Centre
University of Essex
Wivenhoe Park
Colchester
Essex CO4 3SQ
Advice line: 01206 873820
Fax: 01206 874026

TAMBA
(Twins and Multiple Births Association)
PO Box 30
Little Sutton
South Wirrel
Liverpool L66 1TH
Tel: 0151 348 0020

Glossary

alexithymia   A difficulty in communicating/expressing emotions

abandoned cycle   A treatment cycle which is cancelled after commencement of drugs but before embryo transfer

adoption   Taking a new person into an existing relationship; legal adoption of a child

adrenal   Pertaining to or produced by the adrenal glands

adrenaline   A hormone secreted by the adrenal glands, affecting circulation and muscular action, and causing excitement and stimulation

adrenocortical hyperdysfunction   A condition in which the adrenal cortex releases too much adrenocorticol hormone

adrenocortical hypodysfunction   A condition in which the adrenal cortex releases too little adrenocorticol hormone

alternative families   Families not conforming to the norm (that is, not conforming to the nuclear family set-up), for social, genetic or legal reasons

altruistic   A descriptive term for the unselfish consideration of others

amenorrhoea   A condition in women in which there is no menstrual cycle

androgens   Male sex hormones

anonymity   A state in which the origin, background or source of something remains unknown

anonymous donors   Donors whose identity remains unknown

anorexia   The prolonged absence of appetite; a condition believed to be induced by emotional disturbances

anti-sperm antibodies   Antibodies developed within the individual which reject the individual's own sperm

anxiety   A state of excessive unease

aroused   In a state of excitement

artificial insemination (AI)   The insemination of sperm into the woman using a syringe

artificial insemination by donor (AID)   AI using donor sperm

artificial insemination by husband (AIH)   AI using the husband's /partner's sperm

artificial reproductive technology (ART)   A collective term for the specialist infertility treatments designed to increase the number of gametes or to bring them closer together, resulting in the improved probability of conception where otherwise it would not be possible

assisted conception unit (ACU)   A clinic specialising in ART treatments

attachment styles   The means of attachment to someone

autoagglutinating   Self-combining or self-adhering

autoimmobilising   Affecting (via antibodies) the movement of sperm

autoimmunisation   Immunisation against a disease, produced naturally in the body as a result of a reaction to invasion of the disease or associated organisms

autosomes   In humans, 22 pairs of non-sex-related chromosomes

basal body temperature (BBT)   The body temperature taken immediately after awakening and used to predict ovulation for the rhythm method of birth control

bereavement   A desolate feeling as a result of the death of a loved one

bio-behavioural   Behavioural and biological interactions and effects

birth mother   The term for a woman who gives birth to a baby (not necessarily conceived by or genetically related to her)

blood hormone levels   The levels of circulating hormones in the bloodstream

bulb of the vestibule   Either of two elongated masses of erectile tissue within the orifice of the vagina and joined in front by the commissure

case history   A continuous and methodical record of events and details (usually medical) concerning an individual

central nervous system   The system comprising the brain and spinal cord

cervicitis   Inflammation of the cervix

cervix   The neck of the uterus, opening to the vagina

chemotherapy   The treatment of a disease, especially cancer, by chemical means

chlamydia   A micro-organism in the genitourinary tract, usually transmitted through sex

chromosome   One of the small parts of a cell containing the genes or DNA. Each cell contains 46 chromosomes: 22 pairs and 2 sex chromosomes

circulating antibodies   Antibodies circulating freely in the body

clinical depression   Depression characterised by strong signs of inability to cope or a morbid state

clitoris   A small erectile organ in the female, partially hidden by the labia minora

cloning   Producing genetically identical (that is, having the same nuclear gene set) individuals

coitus interruptus   Sex in which the penis is withdrawn from the vagina before ejaculation takes place

commercial surrogacy   Surrogacy carried out as a business venture, characterised by financial gain

commissioning mother   The woman instructing another to carry a baby, who usually provides payment for the act

commodification   The transformation of things into goods, obtained through trade

conception   The act of becoming pregnant, conceiving

confidential register   A register for the purposes of keeping information secret

confidentiality   The full assurance of trust that information provided in confidence will not be revealed

congenital   The term describing conditions, malformations or deformities which are present at birth or discovered soon after birth

consent   Permission from the recipient for treatment to proceed. Consent must be 'informed'

contraceptive   Any agent or method used to prevent conception

coping styles   Methods of coping with life or specific situations in life

corpus luteum   The 'yellow body' which develops into the ovarian follicle after an ovum is produced. It secretes progesterone

cortisol   Hydrocortisone; a naturally occurring glucocorticoid secreted by the adrenal glands

counselling   The process in which specialists help individuals to cope with various situations in their lives

cryopreserved   Preserved by freezing

delayed childbearing   Leaving childbearing until a later age

deoxyribonucleic acid (DNA)   A chemical substance that is responsible for passing hereditary characteristics from parent to offspring

depression   A state of morbidly excessive melancholy or hopelessness

diabetes   A disease of which there are many forms, characterised by a high fasting blood sugar level, an exaggerated rise in the blood sugar level after the ingestion of glucose, and a failure of the blood sugar level to return to a normal level in a reasonable time

diagnosis   A term referring to the identification of a disease or condition from which a person suffers by means of its signs or symptoms; a statement or conclusion drawn from such an analysis

dilation and curettage (D & C)   A relatively minor surgical procedure in which the cervix is dilated to allow the uterine wall to be scraped with a curette

disclosure   The revealing of origins or sources

discontinued treatment   Treatment which has been stopped

dispositional   Relating to temperament, natural tendency or inclination

donor insemination (DI)   A procedure in which sperm is donated (usually anonymously), from a man who is not the woman's husband or partner, and inserted into the woman

donors   Persons providing their gametes (eggs or sperm) for use by another

douching   Applying a stream of liquid at moderate pressure, via a tube, into a body cavity through a natural orifice (for example, the vagina)

dysfunction   Impaired or abnormal functioning

dysmenorrhea   A condition characterised by severe menstrual pain, associated with abdominal cramping and back- and leg-ache

early menopause   Menopause starting at a much earlier age than normal

egg collection   The procedure in which egges are collected from the ovaries using an ultrasound-guided needle or laparoscope; also known as egg harvesting or egg retrieval

egg sharing   The practice in which one woman's eggs are collected and shared with another woman undergoing similar treatment

ejaculate   The seminal fluid expelled during ejaculation

ejaculation   The emission of seminal fluid at orgasm

embryo   The term for a fertilised egg at up to eight weeks' development

embryo reduction   A process in which one or more embryos is chosen to die through medical intervention in order to increase the chances of survival for the remaining embryo(s)

embryo transfer (ET)   The transfer of one or more embryos to the uterus

endocrine system   The collective term for the hormone-producing glands

endometriosis   A condition in which endometrial tissue is present in abnormal situations in the body

endometrium   The lining of the womb

erectile disorder   A sexual disorder in a man characterised by an inability to control an erection

erection   The term for an enlarged or erect penis

ethical   Relating to moral principles or rules of conduct

ethics committee   A committee which oversees the ethical considerations relating to proposed treatments, to research, to patients or to methods, usually consisting of several people

ethnic background   A person's racial, religious, cultural, and so on, origins

fallopian tube   The long narrow tube between an ovary and the uterus, which transports the egg from the ovary to the uterus

fecundity   Fertility

female orgasmic disorder   A disorder characterised by a persistent or recurrent delay or absence of orgasm

fertilisation   The term describing the penetration of the ovum by sperm

fertility   The ability to produce offspring

fertility index   A measure of live births

fibroids   Fibrous tissue in the uterus

fimbriae   Tubes bordered with hairs

foetal reduction   The surgical reduction in the the number of foetuses inside the uterus. This procedure is used following ovarian stimulation with fertility drugs if the number of foetuses is considered to be too high and likely to reduce the chances of healthy babies being produced

foetus   The term used to describe an embryo after eight weeks' development and until birth

follicle   A small sac in the ovary in which the egg develops

follicle stimulating hormone (FSH)   A hormone which stimulates the ovaries or testes

fostering   The process involving the provision by an adult of a caring or nurturing relationship with a child who is not usually genetically related

gamete   The female egg or male sperm

gamete intrafallopian transfer (GIFT)   A procedure in which eggs are collected from the ovaries and returned to the fallopian tubes with a sperm sample for fertilisation to take place as naturally as possible

general anaesthetic   Anaesthetic that affects the whole body

genetic link   A link resulting from the assured biological relatedness of one person to another

genetic parents   Parents who are both genetically related to a child

genetic surrogacy   Surrogacy in which the surrogate mother uses her own genetic material (her gamete) in the conception of a child relinquished at birth

genitourinary   Of or relating to the genital and urinary organs and their functions

German measles   Rubella

gestation   The period during which the baby is carried in the womb

gestational surrogacy   Surrogacy in which the surrogate or carrying mother gestates an unrelated embryo which is relinquished at birth to its genetic parents

glands   Organs secreting substances in the body

GnRH (gonadotropin releasing hormone) agonist   A drug which prevents the working of the body's normal ovulatory controls

gonadal dysgenesis   Incomplete or defective development of the gonads

gonads   Reproductive glands producing gametes

gonadotropins   Pituitary hormones that stimulate the reproductive system

gonorrhea   A venereal disease characterised by inflammatory discharge from the urethra or vagina

graafian follicle   A small sac in the ovary in which ova mature

granulosa cells   Small cells

grieving   The process of coping emotionally with the loss of a loved one

grounded theory   Theory following reflexive methodology, using unstated assumptions and privileged subjectivity

gynaecology   The branch of medicine concerned with the reproductive system

hepatitis B   Serum hepatitis

history   A continuous methodical record of events (usually medical)

hormones   Chemicals secreted by the endocrine system into the bloodstream to be transported to the tissue on which they act

human immunodeficiency virus (HIV)   Any of a group of retroviruses that infect and destroy helper T cells of the immune system; HIV causes AIDS

hypoplasia   The defective formation or underdevelopment of tissue or a bodily part

hypospadias   A congenital defect of the wall of the male urethra or the female vagina, so that instead of the normal external orifice there is an opening of a greater or lesser size on the underside of the penis or vagina

hypothyroidism   A condition caused by underactivity of the thyroid gland; thyroid deficiency

identifying information   Any information that reveals origins or details about a person

immunologic incompatibility   The term used to describe the rejection by one person's immune system of cells from another person, through the development of antibodies

implications counselling   Counselling which focuses on discussion of the implications of diagnosis or treatment for an individual or others affected

impotence   The term used to describe a man's inability to achieve or maintain an erection

incomplete genomic imprinting   Genomic imprinting which has not been completed

incubator   The endometrial lining of the womb, which in normal conditions allows a foetus to be carried to term

in-depth interviews   Thorough and usually lengthy interviews involving two or more people

infertility   The inability to produce offspring

informed consent   Consent based on adequate information

infundibulum   The widening end-part of the fallopian tube

intrauterine insemination (IUI)   A procedure in which the ova are stimulated with drugs and sperm is inserted into the uterus via a catheter

intracytoplasmic sperm injection (ICSI)   A procedure in which a single sperm is injected directly into an egg

in vitro fertilisation (IVF)   A procedure in which an egg is fertilised outside the body, in a petri dish

isolating genes   A strategy for studying mitochondrial structure and function by isolating and mapping nuclear genes

Klinefelter's syndrome   A physical and behavioural condition associated with an XYY chromosome pattern

known donor   A donor who is known to the recipient of that donor's donated material

labia majora and minora   The lips of the female pudenda. The labia majora are the outer folds, the labia minora the inner folds

laparoscopy   A procedure in which a tube is inserted into the abdominal cavity to determine the condition of the pelvis, tubes, ovaries and womb

laparotomy   An exploratory procedure involving an incision into the peritoneal cavity for diagnostic purposes

legal parents   Persons who are the recognised parents of a child by law. They are not necessarily genetically related to the child

licence   A document giving permission or authorisation for a specific action

life event   An important event in a person's life

live birth rate   The number of live births achieved per 100 treatment cycles

lumbar sympathectomy   A technique for the treatment of chronic ischaemia (inadequate or blocked blood supply)

luteinising hormone (LH)   A hormone that stimulates the pituitary gland to produce gonadotropins

maladjustment   Inappropriate adjustment

male orgasmic disorder   A disorder characterised by a persistent or recurrent delay or absence of orgasm

malpractice   Maltreatment; faulty treatment

marital maladjustment   Unhappiness and dissatisfaction with the marital situation

masturbation   The production of sexual orgasm by manual stimulation of the genitals

menopause   The period in a woman's life marked by final cessation of menses

menorrhagia   Prolonged menstrual bleeding

menses or menstruation   The blood loss occurring at the end of the menstrual cycle if pregnancy has not occurred

menstrual cycle   A cycle of approximately 28 days in the female during which an egg is released from an ovary, the uterus swells to receive a fertilised egg and blood is lost from the uterus if pregnancy does not occur

micromanipulation   Any technique used in fertilisation treatment to bypass the zona pellucida surrounding the egg

microsurgical epididymal sperm aspiration (MESA)   A technique that involves inserting a fine needle into the epididymis and extracting a small sample of semen

miscarriage   The spontaneous loss of a foetus before 24 weeks

mitochondrial   Of or relating to the filamentous rod-shaped organelles, found in the cytoplasm of respiring cells enclosed by an outer and inner mitochondrial membrane

monitoring   Observing, listening to and reporting; maintaining regular surveillance

mons pubis   The superficial cushion of fat covering the body of the pubis

morality   Moral science; moral principles; points of ethics

multiple pregnancies   More than one pregnancy; more than one foetus

mumps   An infectious disease caused by a virus. In post-pubertal males, orchitis (inflammation of the testes) complications can arise

myomas   Benign tumours composed of muscle elements

myometrium   The muscular mass of the uterus

neuroendocrine   Relating to hormonal substances that influence the activity of nerves

non-identifying information   Information which does not reveal origins, or details about a person

nuclear family   A family comprising two adults sharing the breadwinning and nurturing functions for the child(ren) living with them

obstetrics   The branch of medicine dealing with birth and its antecedents and sequels

oestrogens   Female sex hormones

oocyte   An egg

orgasm   The climax of sexual excitement

orgasmic disorder   A persistent or recurrent delay or absence of orgasm

ovum (pl. **ova**)   A female germ cell (egg) capable of developing into a new individual when fertilised by a male sperm

ovarian failure   The failure in functioning of the ovaries

ovarian function   The functioning of the ovaries

ovarian hyperstimulation syndrome (OHSS)   A syndrome in which the ovaries react to drugs by overproducing follicles, thus endangering the health of the woman; a possible serious side-effect of treatment

ovaries   The female reproductive glands situated on either side of the uterus, connected by the fallopian tubes. Here the egg cells develop into follicles, and oestrogen and progesterone are produced

ovulation   The term for the release of the ripened oocyte from the ovarian follicle

Parental Order   A regulation allowing parental rights and obligations to be transferred from the surrogate or birth parent(s) to the commissioning parents

parous   The term used to describe a woman who has given birth

patient satisfaction   A feeling of satisfaction with treatment or the environment in which the patient is treated

pelvic inflammatory disease (PID)   A common cause of tubal infection, also involving the ovaries and peritoneum

penis   The sex and urinary organ of the male

perineum   The region of the body between the anus and the vulva or scrotum

pituitary   A gland at the base of the brain which releases FSH and LH

polycystic disease   A condition in which a large number of ovarian cysts prevent fertility

polyps   Tumours with stalks arising from mucous membranes or the surface of the body

post-adoption   Following the adoption of a child

post-coital   Following coitus or sex

post-coital test (PCT)   A test conducted after sex to assess the interaction of the spermatozoa and mucus

posterior urethral stricture   An abnormal narrowing of the urethra

pre-conception   Prior to conception

pre-embryo   A term for the stage of development before the embryonic state

preimplantation genetic diagnosis (PGD)   The term for numerous techniques used to detect genetic abnormalities in an embryo prior to implantation

premature ejaculation   Emission of the seminal fluid at the beginning of sex

premenstrual symptoms   Symptoms such as back-ache and leg-ache, irritability, nausea and tension, associated with the premenstrual or late luteal phase of the menstual cycle

prenatal   Before birth

primary infertility   Infertility in a woman who has never had a pregnancy

progestins   Progestational hormones, involved in preparing the female body for pregnancy

prognosis   The forecast or likely course of disease

promiscuity   Having regular sexual relations not limited by marriage or cohabitation; (casual) sex with others

pronatalism   The term for the subscription to procreation

prospective study   A study investigating events as they occur. These are often longitudinal follow-up studies

prostatitis   A condition in which the prostate is inflamed as a result of infection

prostatectomy   A procedure involving the excision of part of or the entire prostate gland

psychoanalytic   Of or relating to the therapeutic method of investigating disorders, drawing on the interactions between conscious and unconscious elements

psychogenic   Originating in the mind

psychological dysfunction   Abnormal or impaired functioning of the psychological processes

public debate   A debate opened up to the public, usually initiated to obtain consensus on an issue

quality of life   The happiness in or value of life

randomised controlled trial (RCT)   A trial in which participants are allocated using random processes in order to study them under one of several conditions

recipient   The term for a woman who receives and egg from another woman during treatment

regulation   The control by rule, subject to restrictions

rehabilitation   The restoration to proper condition or effectiveness through specific training

relinquishment   The giving up or abandonment of something

repeated failure   Treatment failure on more than one occasion

research   Careful search or inquiry; to discover facts by the scientific study of a subject using a prescribed course of action or method

resolution   The act of causing a discordant state to pass into a concordant state

ribonucleic acid (RNA)   A nucleic acid that plays an essential role in the synthesis of proteins

scrotum   The bag containing the testicles

secondary infertility   Infertility in a woman who has had a previous pregnancy but not necessarily a delivery

semen   The fluid of the ejaculate which contains the sperm and secretions

sexual arousal disorder   A disorder characterised by difficulty or inability to become or remain sexually aroused

sexual aversion disorder   A condition peculiar to women which is characterised by a strong aversion to genital contact

social stigma   Social disgrace as a result of society's unacceptance of an individual's behaviour

social support   Support received from other people important to the individual

somatic conditions   Physical conditions; conditions manifesting themselves in the body

sperm or spermatozoon (pl. **spermatozoa**)   The developed male reproductive cell

spontaneous pregnancies   Pregnancies occurring naturally, without planning or intervention

sterility   An unfruitful or unreproductive state; permanent infertility

stigma   The spot on the surface of an ovary indicating the site of future rupture of a graafian follicle

subfertility   Describes the delay in producing offspring due to problems with conceiving

subzonal insemination (SUZI)   A procedure in which sperm is inserted into the space between the zona pellucida and the egg cell's membrane

superovulation   The production of as many as 30 eggs in any one cycle using drug treatment. Normal ovulation produces one egg per cycle

supportive counselling   Counselling involved with supporting individuals with specific problems

surrogacy   The process involving a woman carrying a baby for another person. Surrogacy is used in the UK only in cases where medical reasons (for example, congenital absence of the womb) indicate this as the only solution to childlessness

surrogate mother   The woman carrying a baby for another person

surrogate pregnancy   A pregnancy for the sole reason of an arrangement between individuals in which the pregnancy will result in a baby for the commissioning mother rather than the surrogate mother

syphilis   A contagious venereal disease initially affecting mainly the skin or mucous membrane of the genitalia, but which can later involve any organ or tissue

test-tube babies   The common name given to babies conceived outside the body through IVF

testes or **testicles**   The two male reproductive organs that are the site of spermatogenesis

testicular germinal aplasia   The term for the defective development of the germinal tissue of the gonads

testicular sperm extraction (TESE)   A procedure similar to MESA, except that a small mount of testicular tissue is removed and the sperm cells are extracted from that tissue

theca cells   The sheath- or envelope-type cells found around the ovaries

therapeutic   Concerned with the treatment of a condition

therapeutic counselling   Counselling which involves helping an individual to cope with investigations and treatments

thyroid   A thyroxine-secreting gland

transportation   The transport of something or a substance from one area to another

transvaginal ultrasound   Ultrasound carried vaginally by the insertion of a camera through the vagina and cervix into the womb

tubal obstructions   Obstructions or blockages of the tubes

tuberculosis (TB)   A disease caused by infection with the myobacterium tuberculosis

ultrasound   A technique using sound waves to produce a picture of the uterus or ovaries. It is used to monitor egg development and foetal growth

undescended testes   A condition in which the testes have failed to descend from the pelvic area

unexplained fertility   The term for infertility where tests on the male or female have been exhausted and no abnormality is detectable, that is, where there is no obvious cause for infertility

unprotected sex   Sex in which methods for preventing pregnancy are not used

unviable   Incapable of sustaining life

uterine abnormalities   Abnormalities of the uterus

uterus   The womb

vagina   The canal between the womb and the external genital area

vaginismus   A condition characterised by painful spasmodic contractions of the vagina

vaginitis   A condition in which the vagina is inflamed

venereal disease   A disease transmitted via sex

vulva   The external female genitals; the external orifice of the vagina

womb   The uterus; the hollow muscular organ where the foetus develops

zona pellucida   The outer covering or layer of an embryo

zygote   A cell formed by the union or joining of two gametes

zygote intrafallopian transfer (ZIFT)   A procedure in which the actual fertilisation of the egg is carried out and confirmed in the laboratory, then the zygote is transferred into the fallopian tube

Bibliography

Allen, K.D., Maguire, K.B., Williams, G.E. and Sanger, W.G. (1996) The effects of infertility on parent–child relationships and adjustment. *Children's Health Care*, 25, 2, 93–105.

Allison, G.H. (1997) Motherhood, motherliness, and psychogenic infertility. *Psychoanalytic Quarterly*, 66, 1, 1–17.

American Fertility Society (1992) *Investigation of the Infertile Couple*. American Fertility Society, Birmingham, AL.

Anonymous (1999) Letter. *CHILDchat*, 83 (Spring), 13.

Applegarth, L., Goldberg, N., Cholst, I. et al. (1995) Families created through ovum donation: A preliminary investigation of obstetrical outcome and psychosocial adjustment. *Journal of Assisted Reproduction and Genetics*, 12, 574–80.

Bahadur, G. (2001) The Human Rights Act (1998) and its impact on reproductive issues. *Human Reproduction*, 16, 4, 785–9.

Balasch, J. (2000) Investigation of the infertile couple. *Human Reproduction*, 15, 11, 2251–7.

Balen, A. (1998) BFS Surrogacy Survey, *Human Fertility*, 1, 6–9.

Baluch, B. (1998) Psychological consequences of infertility. *The Psychologist*, 11, 10, 495.

Bancroft, I. (1983) *Human Sexuality and it's Problems*. Churchill Livingstone, Edinburgh.

Band, D.A., Edelmann, R.J., Avery, S. and Brinsden, P. (1998) Correlates of psychological distress in relation to male infertility. *British Journal of Health Psychology*, 1, 245–56.

Baram, D., Tourtelot, E., Muechler, E. and Huang, K. (1988) Psychosocial adjustment following unsuccessful in vitro fertilization. *Journal of Psychosomatic Obstetrics and Gynaecology*, 9, 181.

Baran, A. and Pannor, R. (1993) *Lethal Secrets. The Psychology of Donor Insemination. Problems and Solutions*, 2nd edn. Amistad, New York.

Bardwick, J. (1974) Evolution and Parenting. *Journal of Social Issues*, 30, 39–62.

Benson, J. and Robinson-Walsh, D. (1998) *Infertility and IVF. Facts and Feelings from Patients' Perspectives*. Scarlet Press, London.

Berger, A. (2001) News roundup. Scientists create first genetically modified monkey. *British Medical Journal*, 322, 128.

Berger, D.M. (1980) Impotence following the discovery of azoospermia. *Fertility and Sterility*, 34, 154–6.

Bertakis, K., Callahan, E., Helms, L., Azari, R., Robbins, J. and Miller, J. (1998) Physician practice styles and patient outcomes: Differences between family practice and general internal medicine. *Medical Care*, 36, 6, 879–91.

Biervliet, F., Maguiness, S., Hay, D., Killick, S. and Atkin, S. (2001) Induction of lactation in the intended mother of a surrogate pregnancy: Case report. *Human Reproduction*, 16, 3, 581–3.

Blank, R. (1990) *Regulating Reproduction*. Columbia University Press, New York.

Blyth, E. (1994) I wanted to be interesting. I wanted to be able to say 'I've done something interesting with my life.' Interviews with surrogate mothers in Britain. *Journal of Reproductive and Infant Psychology*, 12, 3, 189–98.

Blyth, E. (1995) 'Not a primrose path': Commissioning parents' experiences of surrogacy arrangements in Britain. *Journal of Reproductive and Infant Psychology*, 13, 3/4, 185–96.

Boivin, J., Andersson, L., Skoog Svanberg, A., Hjelmstedt, A., Collins, A. and Bergh, T. (1998) Psychological reactions during in-vitro fertilization: Similar response patterns in husbands and wives. *Human Reproduction*, 13, 11, 3262–7.

Botting, B. et al. (eds) (1990) *Three, Four or More. A Study of Triplets and Higher Order Births*. HMSO, London.

Bourguignon, O., Navelet, C. and Fourcault, D. (1998) Psychological study of 20 women after failed in vitro fertilization attempts. *Contraception fertilite Sexualite*, 26, 9, 673.

Bowlby, J. (1969) *Attachment*. Hogarth Press, London.

Braeways, A. (2001) Parent–child relationships and child development in donor insemination families. *Human Reproduction Update*, 7, 38–46.

Branigan, T. and Carter, H. (2001) Controversy rages over the twins sold to highest bidder. *Guardian*, 17 January.

Brazier, M., Golombok, S. and Campbell, A. (1997) *Surrogacy: Review for the UK Health Ministers of Current Arrangements for Payments and Regulation*. Consultation document and questionnaire. Department of Health, London.

British Medical Association (BMA) (1996) *Changing Conceptions of Motherhood. The Practice of Surrogacy in Britain*. BMA, London.

British Medical Journal (BMJ) (2001) STI's at highest level in UK since 1990. *British Medical Journal* News Extra, 322, 10.

Brodzinski, D., Schechter, M. and Henig, R. (1992) *Being Adopted: The Lifelong Search for Self*. Doubleday, New York.

Brodzinsky, D.M. (1987) Adjustment to adoption: a psychological perspective. *Clinical Psychology Review*, 7, 25–47.

Bron, M.S. and Salmon, J.W. (1998) Infertility services and managed care. *American Journal of Managed Care*, 4, 5, 715–20.

Brook, L., Hedges, S., Jowell, R. and Lewis, J. (1992) *British Social Attitudes: Cumulative Sourcebook – The First Six Surveys*. Gower, Aldershot.

Bryan, E.M. (1992) *Twins and Higher Multiple Births. A Guide to their Nature and Nurture*. Edward Arnold, Sevenoaks.

Chandra, A. and Stephen, E.H. (1998) Impaired fecundity in the United States: 1982–1995. *Family Planning Perspectives*, 30, 1, 34–42.

Chennells, P. and Hammond, C., revised by Lord, J. (1998) *Adopting a Child. New Edition: A Guide for People Interested in Adoption*. BAAF, London.

Christie, B. (1999) News: Patients asked to judge quality of care they receive in hospital. *British Medical Journal*, 319, 7212.

Christie, G.L. (1998) Some socio-cultural and psychological aspects of infertility. *Human Reproduction*, 13, 1, 232–41.

Clamar, A. (1984) Sexual issues and the forensic psychologist. Artificial insemination by donor: The anonymous pregnancy. *American Journal of Forensic Psychology*, 2, 1, 27–37.

Code of Practice of the Human Fertilisation and Embryology Act (1993) Revised version. London.

Colpin, H., DeMunter, A. and Vandemeulebroecke, L. (1998) Parenthood motives in IVF mothers. *Journal of Psychosomatic Obstetrics and Gynaecology*, 19, 1, 19–27.

Connolly, K., Edelmann, R., Bartlett, H., Cooke, I., Lenton, E. and Pike, S. (1993) An evaluation of counselling for couples undergoing treatment for in-vitro fertilization. *Human Reproduction*, 8, 1332–8.

Conrad, R., Schilling, G., Langenbuch, M., Haidl, G. and Liedtke, R. (2001) Alexithymia in male infertility. *Human Reproduction*, 16, 3, 587–92.

Cooke, I.D., Salaiman, R.A., Lenton, E.A. and Parsons, R.J. (1981) Fertility and infertility statistics: Their importance and application. *Clinical Obstetrics and Gynaecology*, 8, 3.

Cotton, K. (1985) *Baby Cotton: For Love or Money*. Dorling Kindersley, London.

Crammond, J. (1998) Counselling needs of patients receiving treatment with gamete donation. *Journal of Community and Applied Social Psychology*, 1, 4, 313–21.

Daniels, K.R. and Taylor, K. (1993) Secrecy and openness in donor insemination. *Politics and the Life Sciences*, 12, 2, 155–70.

Daniluk, J.C. (1996) When treatment fails: The transition to biological child-lessness for infertile women. *Women and Therapy*, 19, 2, 81–98.

Department of Health and Social Security (DHSS) (1984) *Report on the Committee of Inquiry into Human Fertilisation and Embryology* (ed. M. Warnock). HMSO, London.

Department of Health and Social Security (1987) *Human Fertilisation and Embryology: A Framework for Legislation*. Cmnd 259. HMSO, London.

Domar, A.D., Broome, A., Zuttermeister, P.C., Seibel, M. and Friedman, R. (1992) The prevalence and predictability of depression in infertile women. *Fertility and Sterility*, 58, 6, 1158–63.

Donchin, A. (1996) Feminist critiques of new infertility technologies: Implications for social policy. *Journal of Medical Philosophy*, 21, 5, 475–98.

Donegan, C. (1994) An assessment of the counselling needs of GIFT recipients: A pilot study. *Journal of Reproductive and Infant Psychology*, 12, 127–30.

Dubois, D. (1987) Preparing applicants in Wandsworth. *Adoption and Fostering*, II, 2, 35–7.

Dudley, M. and Neave, G. (1997) Issues for families and children where conception was achieved using donor gametes, in Lorbach, C. (ed.) *Let the Offspring Speak: Discussions on Donor Conception*. Donor Conception Support Group of Australia, New South Wales, pp.125–6.

Dutton, G. (1997) *A Matter of Trust: The Essential Guide to Gestational Surrogacy*. Clouds Publishing, California.

Edelmann, R.J. (1990) Emotional aspects of in vitro fertilization procedures: Review. *Journal of Reproductive and Infant Psychology*, 8, 161–73.

Edelmann, R.J. and Connolly, K.J. (1986) Psychological aspects of infertility. *British Journal of Medical Psychology*, 59, 209–19.

Edelmann, R.J. and Connolly, K.J. (1998) Psychological state and psychological strain in relation to infertility. *Journal of Community and Applied Social Psychology*, 1, 4, 303–11.

Edelmann, R.J., Cooke, I.D. and Robson, J. (1992) The impact of infertility on psychological functioning. *Journal of Psychosomatic Research*, 36, 5, 459–68.

Edwards, R. (1989) *Life Before Birth: Reflections on the Embryo Debate.* Hutchinson, London.

Eisenberg, V.H. and Schenker, J.G. (1998) Pre-embryo donation: ethical and legal aspects. *International Journal of Gynecology and Obstetrics*, 60, 1, 51–7.

Ericson, A. and Kallen, B. (2001) Congenital malformations in infants born after IVF: A population based study. *Human Reproduction*, 16, 3, 504–9.

European Society for Human Reproduction and Endocrinology (ESHRE) Capri Workshop (1996) Guidelines to the prevalence, diagnosis, treatment and management of infertility. *Human Reproduction*, 11, 1775–807.

European Society for Human Reproduction and Endocrinology (ESHRE) Preimplantation Genetic Diagnosis (PGD) Consortium Steering Committee (2000) Data collection II (May). *Human Reproduction*, 15, 12, 2673–83.

Fanshel, D., Finch, S. and Grundy, J. (1989) Modes of exit from foster family care and adjustment at time of departure of children with unstable life histories. *Child Welfare*, 68, 391–402.

Fazal, A. (2000) UK Government approves limited cloning of human embryos. *British Medical Journal*, 321, 527.

Fein, E. (1991) Issues in foster family care: Where do we stand? *American Journal of Orthopsychiatry*, 61, 4, 578–83.

Fein, E., Maluccio, A., Hamilton, J. and Ward, D. (1983) After foster care: Outcomes of permanency planning for children. *Child Welfare*, 62, 485–562.

Fertility Nursing Group/Human Fertilisation and Embryology Authority (HFEA) (1990) Human Fertilisation and Embryology *Code of Practice.* London.

Festinger, T. (1983) *No One Ever Asked Us. A Postscript to Foster Care.* Columbia University Press, New York.

Foucault, M. (1976) *The History of Sexuality, Volume 1, An Introduction.* Editions Gallimard/Penguin Books Ltd, London.

Freeman, E.W., Rickels, K., Tausig, J., Boxer, A., Mastroianni, L. and Tureck, R.W. (1987) Emotional and psychosocial factors in follow up of women after IVF-ET treatment. *Acta Obstetrica et Gynecologica Scandinavica*, 66, 517–21.

Gennaro, S., Klein, A. and Miranda, L. (1992) Health Policy dilemmas related to high technology infertility services. *Image: Journal of Nursing Scholarship*, 24, 3, 191–4.

Gerrits, T. (1997) Social and cultural aspects of infertility in Mozambique. *Patient Education and Counselling*, 31, 1, 39–48.

Gianaroli, L., Plachot, M., van Kooi, R. et al. (2000) ESHRE guidelines for good practice in IVF laboratories. *Human Reproduction*, 15, 10, 2241–6.

Gilling-Smith, C., Smith, J. and Semprini, A. (2001) Editorial. HIV and infertility: Time to treat. *British Medical Journal*, 322, 566–7.

Glatstein, I, Harlow, B and Hornstein, M (1997) Practice patterns among reproductive endocrinologists: The infertility evaluation. *Fertility and Sterility*, 67, 443–51.

Glatstein, I., Harlow, B. and Hornstein, M. (1998) Practice patterns among reproductive endocrinologists: Further aspects of the infertility evaluation. *Fertility and Sterility*, 70, 263–9.

Golombok, S., Bhanji, F., Rutherford, T. and Winston, R. (1990) Psychological development of children of the new reproductive technologies: Issues and a pilot study of children conceived by IVF. *Journal of Reproductive and Infant Psychology*, 8, 1, 37–43.

Golombok, S., Murray, C., Brinsden, P. and Abdalla, H. (1999) Social versus biological parenting: Family functioning and the socioemotional development of children conceived by egg or sperm donation. *Journal of Child Psychology and Psychiatry*, 40, 519–27.

Gordon, E. (1992) *Mommy, Did I Grow in Your Tummy? Where Some Babies Come From*. Em Greenberg, Santa Monica, CA.

Gottlieb, C., Lalos, O. and Lindblad, F. (2000) Disclosure of donor inseminations to the child: The impact of Swedish legislation on couples' attitudes. *Human Reproduction*, 15, 9, 2052–6.

Greenfield, D. (1997) Infertility and assisted reproductive technology: The role of the perinatal social worker. *Social Work in Health Care*, 24, 3–4, 39–46.

Greenfield, D., Diamond, M. and DeCherney, A. (1988) Grief reactions following in-vitro fertilization. *Journal of Psychosomatic Obstetrics and Gynaecology*, 8, 169–74.

Greenfield, D. and Haseltine, F. (1986) Candidate selection and psychosocial consideration of in vitro fertilization procedures. *Clinical Obstetrics and Gynaecology*, 29, 119–26.

Guerra, D., Llobera, A., Veiga, A. and Barri, P.N. (1998) Psychiatric morbidity in couples attending a fertility service. *Human Reproduction*, 13, 6, 1733–6.

Hajal, F. and Rosenberg, E.B. (1991) The family life cycle in adoptive families. *American Journal of Orthopsychiatry*, 61, 78–85.

Hall, S. (2000) Gay pair plan their third baby. *Guardian*, 1 June.

Halman, L., Abbey, A. and Andrews, F. (1992) Attitudes about infertility interventions among fertile and infertile couples. *American Journal of Public Health*, 82, 2, 191–4.

Halman, L.J., Oakley, D. and Lederman, R. (1995) Adaptation to pregnancy and motherhood among subfecund and fecund primiparous women. *Maternal-Child Nursing Journal*, 23, 3, 90–100.

Hammarberg, K., Astbury, J. and Baker, H. (2001) Women's experience of IVF: A follow-up study. *Human Reproduction*, 16, 2, 374–83.

Hardy, G., West, M. and Hill, D. (1996) Components and predictors of patient satisfaction. *British Journal of Health Psychology*, 1, 1, 65–85.

Harrison, R.F., O'Moore, A.M., O'Moore, R.R. and Robb, D. (1984) Stress in infertile couples, in Bunnar, J. and Thomson, W. (eds) *Fertility and Sterility*. MTP Press, Lancaster.

Helmerhorst, F., Oei, S. and Keirse, M. (1997) Clinical tutorial in evidence-based medicine: The prognostic value of the postcoital test. Abstract no. O-099. *Human Reproduction*, 12 (Abstract Book 1), 47.

Hill, M., Lambert, L. and Triseliotis, J. (1989) *Achieving Adoption with Love and Money*. National Children's Bureau, London.

Hill, M., and Shaw, M. (1998) *Signposts in Adoption*. BAAF, London.

Hobbins, J.C. (1988) Selective reduction – a perinatal necessity? *New England Journal of Medicine*, 318, 1062–3.

Hobday, A.M. and Lee, K. (1995) Adoption: A specialist area for psychology? *The Psychologist* (January), 13–15.

Hoffman, L. and Hoffman, M. (1973) The value of children to parents, in Fawcett, J.T. (ed.) *Psychological Perspectives on Population*. Basic Books, New York.

Holcomb, W., Parker, J., Leong, G., Thiele, J. and Higdon, J. (1998) Customer satisfaction and self-reported measurement outcomes among psychiatric inpatients. *Psychiatric Services*, 49, 7, 929–34.

Holloway, R. (1999) *Godless Morality: Keeping Religion Out of Ethics*. Canongate Books Ltd, Edinburgh, pp.131–49.

Houghton, P. (1984) Infertility: The consumer's outlook. *British Journal of Sexual Medicine*, 11, 185–7.

Howe, D. (1996) *Adopters on Adoption: Reflections on Parenthood and Children*. BAAF, London.

Howe, D. and Feast, J. (2000) *Adoption, Search and Reunion. The Long Term Experience of Adopted Adults*. The Children's Society, London.

Howe, D., Sawbridge, P. and Hinings, D. (1997) *Half a Million Women: Mothers who Lose their Children by Adoption*. BAAF, London.

Human Fertilisation and Embryology Authority (HFEA) (1990) *Code of Practice*. HFEA, London.

Human Fertilisation and Embryology Authority (1991) HFEA, London.

Human Fertilisation and Embryology Authority (1992) *Annual Report*. HFEA, London.

Human Fertilisation and Embryology Authority (1993) *Code of Practice*. HFEA, London.

Human Fertilisation and Embryology Authority (1996) HFEA, London.

Humphrey, M. (1984) Infertility and alternative parenting, in Broome, A. and Wallace, L.M. (eds) *Psychology and Gynaecological Problems*. Tavistock, London.

ICM Research (1994) *Results of a Poll on Infertility Treatment Conducted for 'The Observer'*. ICM, London.

Jennings, S.E. (ed.) (1995) *Infertility Counselling*. Blackwell Science, Oxford.

Jewett, C.L. (1995) *Helping Children Cope with Separation and Loss*. The Harvard Common Press, Boston, MA.

Josefson, D. (2000) News: Couple select healthy embryo to provide stem cells for sister. *British Medical Journal*, 321, 917.

Khanna, J., Van Look, P. and Griffin, P. (1992) *Reproductive Health: A Key to a Brighter Future.* WHO, Geneva.

Kline, D. and Overstreet, H. (1972) *Foster Care of Children: Nurture and Treatment.* Columbia University Press, New York.

Kol, S. and Itskovitz-Eldor, J. (2000) Severe OHSS. Yes, there is a strategy to prevent it! *Human Reproduction*, 15, 11, 2266–7.

Kon, A. (1993) Infertility: The real costs. *Issue*, Birmingham.

Langdridge, D., Connolly, K. and Sheeran, P. (2000) Reasons for wanting a child: A network analytic study. *Journal of Reproductive and Infant Psychology*, 18, 4, 321–38.

Lansac, J. and Royere, D. (2001) Follow-up studies of children born after frozen sperm donation. *Human Reproduction Update*, 7, 33–7.

Lawson, K. (2001) Contemplating selective reproduction: The subjective appraisal of parenting a child with a disability. *Journal of Reproductive and Infant Psychology*, 19, 1, 73–82.

Leiblum, S. and Aviv, A. (1998) Disclosure issues and decisions of couples who conceived via donor insemination. *Journal of Psychosomatic Obstetrics and Gynaecology*, 18, 4, 292–300.

Leiblum, S.R., Kemmann, E. and Lane, M.K. (1987) The psychological concomitants of in vitro fertilization. *Journal of Psychosomatic Obstetrics and Gynaecology*, 6, 165.

Levin, J.B., Sher, T.G. and Theodos, V. (1997) The effect of intracouple coping concordance on psychological and marital distress in infertility patients. *Journal of Clinical Psychology in Medical Settings*, 4, 4, 361–72.

Link, P.W. and Darling, C.A. (1986) Couples undergoing treatment for infertility: Dimensions of life satisfaction. *Journal of Sex and Marital Therapy*, 12, 46–59.

Llewellyn, A., Stowe, Z. and Nemeroff, C. (1997) Depression during pregnancy and the puerperium. *Journal of Clinical Psychiatry*, 58, Supplement 15, 26–32.

Lockwood, G. (1996) The provision of fertility treatment: Implications for parents, children and society. Paper presented at the Royal Society of Medicine Conference on Assisted Fertilisation and it's Social, Legal and Ethical Dilemmas, 3–4 October, London.

Lord, J., Barker, S. and Cullen, D. (1997) *Effective Panels.* BAAF, London.

Mao, K. and Wood, C. (1984) Barriers to treatment of infertility by in-vitro fertilization and embryo transfer. *Medical Journal of Australia*, 28 (April), 532–3.

McLeod, M. (2000) Gay fathers back off surrogacy. *Guardian*, 15 May.

Mahlstedt, P.P. (1985) The psychological component of infertility. *Fertility and Sterility*, 43, 3, 335–46.

Mahlstedt, P.P., MacDuff, S, and Bernstein, J. (1987) Emotional factors and the in vitro fertilization and embryo transfer process. *Journal of In Vitro Fertilization and Embryo Transfer*, 4, 232.

Major, S. (2000) WHO links with consumers on reproductive health information. *British Medical Journal*, 320, 787.

Marsh, M. and Ronner, W. (1996) *The Empty Cradle: Infertility in America from Colonial Times to the Present.* Johns Hopkins University Press, Baltimore, MD.

Masters, W.H. and Johnson, V.E. (1970) *Human Sexual Inadequacy.* Little, Brown, Boston, MA.

Masters, W.H., Johnson, V.E. and Kolodny, R. (1992) *Human Sexuality*, 4th edn. HarperCollins Publishers, New York.

Menning, B.E. (1980) The emotional needs of infertile couples. *Fertility and Sterility*, 34, 313–19.

Menning, B.E. (1982) The psychosocial impact of infertility. *Nursing Clinics of North America*, 17, 1, 155–63.

Miall, C. (1994) Community constructs of involuntary childlessness: Sympathy, stigma, and social support. *Canadian Review of Sociology and Anthropology*, 31, 4, 392–421.

Mikulincer, M., Horesh, N., Levy-Shiff, R., Manovich, R. and Shalev, J. (1998) The contribution of adult attachment style to the adjustment to infertility. *British Journal of Medical Psychology*, 71, 265–80.

Milad, M.P., Klock, S.C., Moses, S. and Chatterton, R. (1998) Stress and anxiety do not result in pregnancy wastage. *Human Reproduction*, 13, 8, 2296–300.

Nachtigall, R.D., Becker, G., Quiroga, S.S. and Tschann, J.M. (1998) The disclosure decision: Concerns and issues of parents of children conceived through donor insemination. *American Journal of Obstetrics and Gynecology*, 199, 6, 1165–8.

Nelson, L. (1998) In Blyth, E., Cranshaw, M. and Speirs, J. (eds) *Truth and the Child 10 Years On: Information Exchange in Donor Assisted Conception.* British Association of Social Workers, Birmingham.

Newton, C.R., Hearn, M.T. and Yuzpe, A.A. (1990) Psychological assessment and follow up after in vitro fertilization: Assessing the impact of failure. *Fertility and Sterility*, 54, 5, 879–86.

Nikolettos, N., Kupker, W., Al-Hasani, S., Demirel, L., Schopper, B., Sturm, R. and Deidrich, K. (2000) ICSI outcome in patients of 40 years and over: A retrospective analysis. *European Journal of Obstetrics and Gynaecologic Reproductive Biology*, 91, 2, 177–82.

O'Gorman, E.C., McBride, M. and McClure, N. (1997) Communication skills training in the area of human sexuality. *Sexual and Marital Therapy*, 12, 4, 377–80.

Olsen, J., Basso, O., Spinelli, A. and Kuppers Chinnow, M. (1998) Correlates of care seeking for infertility treatment in Europe – Implications for health services and research. *European Journal of Public Health*, 8, 1.

Page, S. (1988) Planning and documentation. Addressing patient needs in a day surgery setting. *AORN Journal*, 47, 2, 526–37.

Pennings, G. (2000) Avoiding multiple pregnancies in ART. Multiple pregnancies: A test case for the moral quality of medically assisted reproduction. *Human Reproduction*, 15, 12, 2466–9.

Pepperell, R., Hudson, B. and Wood, C. (1980) *The Infertile Couple.* Churchill Livingstone, Edinburgh.

Persaud, R.N. and Lam, R.W. (1998) Manic reaction after induction of ovulation with gonadotropins. *American Journal of Psychiatry*, 155, 3, 447–8.

Ragone, H. (1994) *Surrogate Motherhood: Conception in the Heart*. Westview Press, Boulder, CO.

Ravin, A., Mahowald, M. and Stocking, C. (1997) Genes or gestation? Attitudes of women and men about biologic ties to children. *Journal of Women's Health*, 6, 6, 639–47.

Reading, A. (1989) Decision making and in-vitro fertilization: The influence of emotional state. *Journal of Psychosomatic Obstetrics and Gynaecology*, 10, 107–12.

Richardson, H. (ed.) (1987) *On the Problem of Surrogate Motherhood: Analysing the Baby M Case*. Symposium series 25. Edwin Mellen, New York/Ontario.

Robinson, G.E. and Steward, D.E. (1996) The psychological impact of infertility and new reproductive technologies. *Harvard Review of Psychiatry*, 4, 3, 168–72.

Rosenfeld, D.L. and Mitchell, E. (1979) Treating the emotional aspects of infertility: Counselling services in an infertility clinic. *American Journal of Obstetrics and Gynecology*, 135, 177–80.

Rosenthal, M. and Goldfarb, J. (1997) Infertility and assisted reproductive technology: An update for mental health professionals. *Harvard Review of Psychiatry*, 5, 3, 167–72.

Rowe, P., Comhaire, F., Hargreave, T. et al. (1993) *WHO Manual for the Standardized Investigation of the Infertile Couple*. Cambridge University Press, Cambridge.

Rutter, M. (1981) *Maternal Deprivation Reassessed* 2nd edn. Penguin, Harmondsworth.

Saban, C. (1998) *Miracle Child: Genetic Mother, Surrogate Womb*. New Horizon Press, Far Hills, NJ.

Sade, R. (1994) Health Care Reform. *Annals of Thorac Surgery*, 57, 4, 792–6.

Safran, D., Taira, D., Rogers, W., Kosinski, M., Ware, J. and Tarlov, A. (1998) Linking primary care performance to outcomes of care. *Journal of Family Practice*, 47, 3, 213–20.

Saleh, A., Tan, S., Biljan, M. and Tulandi, T. (2000) A randomized study of the effect of 10 minutes of bed rest after intrauterine insemination. *Fertility and Sterility*, 74, 3, 509–11.

Sants, H.J. (1964) Genealogical bewilderment in children with substitute parents. *British Journal of Medical Psychology*, 37, 133–41.

Saunders, K. and Bruce, N. (1997) A prospective study of psychosocial stress and fertility in women. *Human Reproduction*, 12, 10, 2324–9.

Schmidt, L. (1998) Infertile couples' assessment of infertility treatment. *Acta Obstetrica et Gynecologica Scandinavica*, 6, 649–53.

Serafini, P. (2001) Outcome and follow-up of children born after IVF-surrogacy. *Human Reproduction Update*, 7, 23–7.

Shalev, C. (1989) *The Case for Surrogacy*. Yale University Press, New Haven, CT.

Shaw, P., Johnston, M. and Shaw, R. (1988) Counselling needs. Emotional and relationship problems in couples awaiting IVF. *Journal of Psychosomatic Obstetrics and Gynaecology*, 9, 171–80.

Sheldon, T. (2000) News: Netherlands bans cloning of human embryos for research. *British Medical Journal*, 321, 854.

Siegel-Itzkovich, J. (2001) News roundup: Israel to allow women to donate their ova. *Human Reproduction*, 322, 816.

Smith, C., Bayley, L., Adhege, J. and van den Akker, O. (2000) Patient satisfaction with assisted conception services: The role of expectations. *Journal of Reproductive and Infant Psychology*, 18, 3, 265.

Snowden, C. (1994) What makes a mother? Interviews with women involved in egg donation and surrogacy. *Birth*, 21, 77–84.

Snowden, R., Mitchell, G. and Snowden, E. (1983) *A Social Investigation*. George Allen and Unwin, London.

Soderstrom-Anttila, V. (2001) Pregnancy and child outcome after oocyte donation. *Human Reproduction Update*, 7, 28–32.

Soderstrom-Anttila, V., Sajaniemi, N., Tiitinen, A. and Hovatta, O. (1998) Health and development of children born after oocyte donation compared with that in those born after in-vitro fertilization, and the parents' attitudes regarding secrecy. *Human Reproduction*, 13, 2009–15.

Spitz, E. (1996) Through her I too shall bear a child: Birth surrogates in Jewish Law. *Journal of Religious Ethics*, 24, 1, 65–97.

Strauss, B., Hepp, U., Staeding, G. and Mettler, L. (1998) Psychological characteristics of infertile couples: Can they predict pregnancy and treatment persistence? *Journal of Community and Applied Social Psychology*, 1, 4, 289–301.

Tabbush, V. and Gambone, J.C. (1998) Managed health care coverage for infertility services: Understanding adverse selection. *Current Opinion in Obstetrics and Gynecology*, 10, 4, 341–6.

Templeton, A. (1996) Factors affecting outcome of assisted reproduction. Paper presented at the Royal Society of Medicine Conference on Assisted Fertilisation and it's Social, Legal and Ethical Dilemmas, 3–4 October, London.

Tesarik, J., Nagy, Z., Mendoza, C. and Greco, E. (2000) Chemically and mechanically induced membrane fusion: Non-activating methods for nuclear transfer in mature human oocytes. *Human Reproduction*, 15, 5, 1149–54.

Triseliotis, J. (1973) *In Search of Origins: The Experiences of Adopted People*. Routledge and Kegan Paul, London.

Triseliotis, J., Sellick, C. and Short, R. (1995) *Foster Care: Theory and Practice*. B.T. Batsford Ltd, London.

Trounson, A. and Wood, C. (1981) Extracorporeal fertilization and embryo transfer. *Clinical Obstetrics and Gynaecology*, 8, 3, 681–713.

Turner, A.J. and Coyle, A. (2000) What does it mean to be a donor offspring? The identity experiences of adults conceived by donor insemination and the implications for counselling and therapy. *Human Reproduction*, 15, 9, 2041–51.

van Balen, F. (1996) Child-rearing following in vitro fertilisation. *Journal of Child Psychology and Psychiatry and Allied Disciplines*, 37, 6, 687–93.

van Balen, F. and Gerrits, T. (2001) Quality of infertility care in poor-resource areas and the introduction of new reproductive technologies. *Human Reproduction*, 16, 2, 215–19.

van Balen, F., Trimbos-Kemper, T. and Verdurmen, J. (1997a) Perception of diagnosis and openness of patients about infertility. *Patient Education and Counselling*, 28, 3, 247–52.

van Balen, F., Verdurmen, J. and Ketting, E. (1997b) Age, the desire to have a child and cumulative pregnancy rate. *Human Reproduction*, 12, 3, 623–7.

van Balen, F., Verdurmen, J. and Ketting, E. (1997c) Choices and motivations of infertile couples. *Patient Education and Counselling*, 31, 1, 19–27.

van den Akker, O.B.A. (1994) Something old, something new, something borrowed, and something taboo. Review article. *Journal of Reproductive and Infant Psychology*, 12, 179–88.

van den Akker, O.B.A. (1998a) Functions and responsibilities of organizations dealing with surrogate motherhood in the UK. *Human Fertility*, 1, 10–13.

van den Akker, O.B.A. (1998b) Motherhood through surrogacy. Paper presented at the British Psychological Society, Psychology for Women Section, 25–27 July, Birmingham.

van den Akker, O.B.A. (1998c) Whose family, what family. British Psychological Society, POWS. Invited paper for 'The Family' symposium, London, 15–16 December.

van den Akker, O.B.A. (1999) Organizational selection and assessment of women entering a surrogacy agreement in the UK. *Human Reproduction*, 14, 1, 101–5.

van den Akker, O.B.A. (2000) The importance of a genetic link in mothers commissioning a surrogate baby in the UK. *Human Reproduction*, 15, 8, 1849–55.

van den Akker, O.B.A. (2001a) Adoption in the age of reproductive technology. *Journal of Reproductive and Infant Psychology*, 19, 2, 147–59.

van den Akker, O.B.A. (2001b) The acceptable face of parenthood: The relative status of biological and cultural interpretations of offspring in infertility treatment. *Psychology, Evolution and Gender*, 3, 2.

van den Akker, O.B.A. (2001c) Coping, quality of life and psychiatric morbidity in 3 groups of subfertile women: Does process or outcome affect psychological functioning? unpublished paper.

van den Akker, O.B.A. (2001d) Psychological Characteristics of British Surrogate Mothers, unpublished paper.

Vercollone, C., Moss, H. and Moss, R. (1997) *Helping the Stork: The Choices and Challenges of Donor Insemination*. Macmillan, New York.

Waller Report (1984) Committee to Consider Social, Ethical and Legal issues arising from in vitro fertilisation, *Report on the Disposition of Embryos Produced by In Vitro Fertilisation*. Parliament of the State of Victoria, Melbourne.

Warnock, M. (1984) *A Question of Life: The Warnock Report on Human Fertility and Embryology*. Blackwell, Oxford.

Watson, R. (2000) News: EU institutions divided on therapeutic cloning. *British Medical Journal*, 321, 658.

Wear, S. (1999) Enhancing clinician provision of informed consent and counselling: Some pedagogical strategies. *Journal of Medical Philosophy*, 24, 1, 34–42.

Weaver, S., Clifford, E., Hay, D. and Robinson, J. (1997) Psychosocial adjustment to unsuccessful IVF and GIFT treatment. *Patient Education and Counselling*, 31, 7–18.

Wheal, A. (1995) *The Foster Carer's Handbook*. Russell House Publishing Ltd, Dorset.

White, G.B. (1998) Crisis in assisted conception: The British approach to an American dilemma. *Journal of Women's Health*, 7, 3, 321–8.

Williams, M.E. (1997) Toward greater understanding of the psychological effects of infertility on women. *Psychotherapy in Private Practice*, 16, 3, 7–26.

Wingfield, M., Wood, C., Henderson, L. and Wood, R. (1997) Treatment of endometriosis involving a self help group positively affects patients' perception of care. *Journal of Psychosomatic Obstetrics and Gynaecology*, 18, 4, 255–8.

Wise, J. (2000) UK lifts ban on frozen eggs. *British Medical Journal*, 320, 334.

World Health Organization (WHO) (1992) Scientific Group on recent advances in medically assisted conception. Geneva, WHO monograph, technical series 820.

Index

Compiled by Sue Carlton